NURSING
BEYOND
THE BEDSIDE

60 NON-HOSPITAL
CAREERS IN NURSING

Susan Eva Lowey, PhD, RN, CHPN

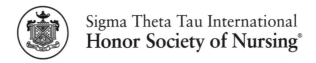

Sigma Theta Tau International
Honor Society of Nursing®

The Honor Society of Nursing, Sigma Theta Tau International (STTI) is a nonprofit organization founded in 1922 whose mission is to support the learning, knowledge, and professional development of nurses committed to making a difference in health worldwide. Members include practicing nurses, instructors, researchers, policymakers, entrepreneurs and others. STTI's 494 chapters are located at 676 institutions of higher education throughout Australia, Botswana, Brazil, Canada, Colombia, Ghana, Hong Kong, Japan, Kenya, Malawi, Mexico, the Netherlands, Pakistan, Portugal, Singapore, South Africa, South Korea, Swaziland, Sweden, Taiwan, Tanzania, United Kingdom, United States, and Wales. More information about STTI can be found online at www.nursingsociety.org.

Sigma Theta Tau International
550 West North Street
Indianapolis, IN, USA 46202

To order additional books, buy in bulk, or order for corporate use, contact Nursing Knowledge International at 888.NKI.4YOU (888.654.4968/US and Canada) or +1.317.634.8171 (outside US and Canada).

To request a review copy for course adoption,
e-mail solutions@nursingknowledge.org or call 888.NKI.4YOU (888.654.4968/US and Canada) or +1.317.634.8171 (outside US and Canada).

To request author information, or for speaker or other media requests, contact Marketing, Honor Society of Nursing, Sigma Theta Tau International at 888.634.7575 (US and Canada) or +1.317.634.8171 (outside US and Canada).

Praise for *Nursing Beyond the Bedside*

"This book is an essential counterbalance to hospital-focused texts in courses introducing students to the profession of nursing. It has the potential to change learners' mental picture of this rich, varied, and highly skilled vocation. As much of healthcare moves outside the acute care setting, Nursing Beyond the Bedside *portrays the essential portability of a well-educated nurse's professional knowledge and contributions. The horizon for nurses in the 21st century is limitless, but to envision a personalized and influential future in nursing requires books such as this one."*

–Margaret H. Kearney, PhD, RN, FAAN
Vice Provost and University Dean of Graduate Studies
Professor, School of Nursing
University of Rochester
Rochester, New York
Editor, *Research in Nursing & Health*

"Kudos to Dr. Lowey for this timely publication, Nursing Beyond the Bedside. *Dr. Lowey does a wonderful job highlighting 60 different roles in nursing. This valuable resource is a must-read for all nurses as it clearly shows that when you are a nurse, the possibilities are endless."*

–Pamela C. Smith, EdD, RN, ANP
Professional Coach, Leadership Consultant, and Educator
President, Class Act Consulting & Professional Development, LLC

"This book is timely as we move into a healthcare era of increased community-based care environments. It is the first text of its kind, focusing on non-hospital nursing care roles. The highlights from nurses practicing in these roles add richness and an appealing picture of practice in community-based settings. Lowey has provided us with a valuable resource for nursing education and for building a strong workforce of nurses in community care settings."

–Tara Hulsey, PhD, RN, CNE, FAAN
Dean and E. Jane Martin Endowed Professor
West Virginia University School of Nursing

ISBN: 9781940446806

EPUB ISBN: 9781940446813

PDF ISBN: 9781940446820

MOBI ISBN: 9781940446837

Library of Congress Cataloging-in-Publication Data

Names: Lowey, Susan Eva, 1972- author.

Title: Nursing beyond the bedside : 60 non-hospital careers in nursing /
    Susan Eva Lowey.

Description: Indianapolis, IN : Sigma Theta Tau International, 2016.

Identifiers: LCCN 2016041027 (print) | LCCN 2016042998 (ebook) | ISBN

    9781940446806 (print : alk. paper) | ISBN 9781940446813 (epub) | ISBN

    9781940446820 (pdf) | ISBN 9781940446837 (mobi) | ISBN
9781940446813

    (Epub) | ISBN 9781940446820 (Pdf) | ISBN 9781940446837 (Mobi)

Subjects: | MESH: Specialties, Nursing | Job Description | Career Choice

Classification: LCC RT82 (print) | LCC RT82 (ebook) | NLM WY 101 | DDC

    610.7306/9--dc23

LC record available at https://lccn.loc.gov/2016041027

Publisher: Dustin Sullivan

Principal Book Editor: Carla Hall

Acquisitions Editor: Emily Hatch

Editorial Coordinator: Paula Jeffers

Copy Editor: Todd Lothery

Cover/Interior Design: TnT Design, Inc.

Proofreader: Todd Lothery

Indexer: Cheryl Lenser

First Printing, 2016

Dedication

I would like to dedicate this book to my husband, Matthew Lowey, who has supported me through all my joys and tears since we first met long ago in 1993. Your encouragement, devotion, and enduring support for all of my good and not-so-good ideas have helped me reach beyond my wildest dreams.

Acknowledgments

There are many people in both my personal and professional life that I would like to give a special acknowledgment to who have helped me throughout my journey to where I am today. First, I would like to thank my mother and father for encouraging me to be whatever I wanted to be. I want to thank my sister, Barb, for always being there for me and supporting me in everything I have done. I would also like to thank my husband, Matt, and my two sons, Erik and Jason, for bearing with me during the process of writing this book and always.

Although I knew I wanted to be a nurse since I was 6 years old, I want to thank Mary Kay Remley, who first introduced me to home health nursing. I applied to her home health agency for a seasonal flu shot clinic position, which was already filled by the time I applied. She offered me another position as a home care nurse, and although I was hesitant at first, I eventually took the job. The knowledge and skills that I learned from her in home care gave me a solid foundation on which I built my nursing career. I also want to give a special thanks to Anne Heeks, who was my supervisor for my first job in hospice nursing. She was the best supervisor I ever had and was always supportive and kind to me.

Since much of my time has been spent as a student as I pursued my graduate education in nursing, I want to thank several of my nursing mentors who have helped me along the way. First, I would like to thank Dr. Dianne Cooney-Miner, Dean of the Wegmans School of Nursing at St. John Fisher College. I would not have ever thought about pursuing my PhD in nursing had it not been for her encouragement, kindness, and support for me as I worked on my master's in nursing in her program. Second, I would like to give a very special thank-you and acknowledgment to Dr. Sally Norton, Associate Professor and Independence Foundation Chair in Nursing and Palliative Care at the University of Rochester, who was my PhD advisor and dissertation chair. I learned so much from her about everything that has led me to where I am today. She taught me more about research and palliative care than any other person I know and was the best role model a doctoral student could have. She was also very supportive to me during a very difficult time in my personal life as I was finishing up the program, and I will forever be grateful to her for that. I would also like to thank Dr. Margaret Kearney, Vice Provost and University Dean of Graduate Studies at the University of Rochester, who was such an influence on me during my doctoral program. I learned so much from her about grant and academic writing, qualitative research, and nursing leadership. She was always willing to help me and all of the other doctoral students who routinely sought her insightful advice. I would also like to extend a thank-you to a few other nursing mentors who had a positive impact on my life: Dr. Bethel Powers, Dr. Jill Quinn, Dr. Dianne Liebel, Dr. Ying Xue, Dr. Judith Baggs, and Dr. Harriet Kitzman.

Lastly, I would like to thank and acknowledge the great group of faculty and staff I currently work with in the Department of Nursing at the State University of New York College at Brockport. There are far too many to individually list here, but I would like to extend a special thank-you to Ms. Patty Sharkey, who recently retired. She was my mentor at Brockport and taught me about academic advisement and all the other important things about being an educator that you can't learn from school. Her outstanding tips and advice will forever be remembered and passed on as I help mentor nursing students, nurses, and new faculty.

About the Author

Susan E. Lowey, PhD, RN, CHPN

An experienced nurse driven by both curiosity and the desire for continual improvement in healthcare and education, Susan E. Lowey, PhD, RN, CHPN, has worked as a clinician, researcher, and educator. She has comforted patients facing the end of life during their darkest hour, methodically executed research studies aimed at improving the care for patients with serious illnesses, and provided encouragement and motivation to students studying to enter the profession. Caring for patients over the past 25 years, Lowey initially began her work in healthcare as a certified nursing assistant. She received her baccalaureate degree in nursing from the State University of New York College at Brockport and her master's degree in nursing as a clinical nurse specialist from St. John Fisher College. She earned her PhD in health practice research from the University of Rochester for her dissertation, focusing on exploring the care preferences of patients with advanced illnesses. She was awarded the prestigious Claire M. Fagin Fellowship from the National Hartford Center of Gerontological Nursing Excellence to support her postdoctoral work. This focused on examining healthcare and opioid utilization during the last year of life among Medicare beneficiaries with advanced illnesses. Currently, Lowey is an Assistant Professor in the Department of Nursing at the State University of New York College at Brockport. She works with both juniors and seniors in the traditional nursing program, teaching community health nursing, nursing research, and nursing care of older adults. Lowey has been awarded several grants that have helped fund her research aimed at improving care for patients at the end of life. She has presented her work at numerous national professional conferences and through peer-reviewed publications. Lowey holds national certification as a board certified hospice and palliative care nurse (CHPN) through the Hospice and Palliative Credentialing Center. In addition, she is a certified ELNEC (end-of-life nursing education consortium) trainer in both core and geriatric care. She is also an appointed member of the Hospice and Palliative Nurses Registered Nurse Examination Development Committee through the Hospice & Palliative Credentialing Center and has been an active member on several committees within the Gerontological Society of America. Lowey has been a member of the Omicron Beta Chapter of the Honor Society of Nursing, Sigma Theta Tau International since 1998 and most recently in the capacity of a chapter counselor since 2012.

Table of Contents

Preface

When I first started teaching the community health course to senior nursing students in our traditional baccalaureate nursing program, I was surprised to find that the majority of students were not aware of the various career opportunities they could pursue outside of the hospital setting. Working as a community-based nurse for years, I wasn't aware that there was such a general lack of knowledge about non-hospital nursing jobs among those studying to enter the profession and among those already working in the profession. I mistakenly assumed that most nurses were aware of these opportunities since my nursing career somehow led me to obtain several nursing positions that were not in the traditional hospital setting. The students' lack of knowledge about this topic fueled my excitement to share the knowledge and passion I have about these non-hospital jobs with nursing students. I began to introduce this topic during the first community health class every semester and even developed a fact sheet for students that included information about the various non-hospital nursing jobs they could pursue after graduation. Board or national certification is another area in nursing professional development that I am passionate about, and I also include information about the certification options that are available with many of these non-hospital nursing specialties.

In my experience as a nurse educator, I have found that many nursing students are not very enamored with community health nursing because most want to work in an acute care inpatient hospital setting. Outside of the misinformation about nursing practice that the average person receives from fictitious television shows focused around a hospital-based theme, I thought about other reasons that influence students to pursue their nursing careers in the hospital. One of these reasons may be due to the fact that the hospital is the most common location of the vast majority of clinical rotations students experience during nursing school. Most baccalaureate nursing programs include a community health or population-focused care course, so nurses graduating with this degree are able to have at least one clinical rotation in an outpatient setting. Clinical experiences in community health are often shorter than other rotations, and students may not be totally immersed in the experience for a variety of factors that are not the focus of this handbook. Secondly, there is an important emphasis in nursing school on the acquisition of technical skills that are requirements to practice as a registered nurse, such as administration of injections or the insertion of catheters. While these skills are important and should most certainly be skills that all nurses possess, there tends to be less of an emphasis on the social aspects of care in general in nursing school. Although nursing students in this country learn about poverty and social injustice to a degree, it is not always experienced by nursing students during their hospital clinical rotations. I wholeheartedly believe that healing requires more than just a restoration of physical health, and in this day and age, medical science can "fix" many diseases and conditions. Due to the various constraints found in the inpatient setting, there is often a lack of time or emphasis that promotes a focus on patients' nonphysical health. This includes patients' psychological, socio-environmental, emotional, and spiritual health and concerns. Since the length and scope of every program may differ in terms of community-based clinical expectations, not all nursing students gain an exposure to the larger societal needs and concerns affecting many patients who are in the hospital setting. It is often difficult for new nurses to see the various determinants of health affecting the broad scope of issues patients have who are in the hospital setting.

I always inform students that while it is imperative to initially work in the hospital to develop experience in nursing knowledge and skills, there are numerous other care settings that they can practice in once they have established a solid foundation in their clinical experience. As you will read in the next section, we are progressing toward a greater need to provide competent, quality, and evidenced-based community care to a growing population in the near future. We will always have hospitals, but their role in healthcare is evolving, and nurses need to be prepared to meet those needs. Every semester, I am happy to see the look of wonder and excitement on many students' faces regarding the endless possibilities that will be waiting for them once they begin their journey in the nursing profession. I have encountered several nursing students who were close to dropping out of the program because they just did not like or enjoy working in the hospital setting. Once they learned about the various non-hospital nursing careers that they could pursue, it changed their outlook, and they had more drive to strive to complete their degree in nursing. It is important that nursing students, practicing nurses, and nurse educators are informed about non-hospital career opportunities so that the profession will be well prepared for the eventual transformation from a predominately acute-care-based to a community-outpatient-oriented healthcare model.

Introduction

Purpose and Description of This Book

The purpose of this book is to introduce nurses and nursing students to the various career opportunities in the field outside of the hospital setting. In order to both attract and retain a competent nursing workforce, it is imperative to showcase the various opportunities for careers within the profession. The profession often loses qualified individuals who have less interest in working at the bedside and are not aware of the other opportunities available for nursing practice. According to the Future of Nursing Initiative from the Robert Wood Johnson Foundation (2008), there is a great need to strengthen the nursing workforce to be able to provide care to a diverse population of patients who are living longer with more chronic illnesses. This is resulting in an ongoing shift in the current healthcare system from predominately acute to community-based. It is imperative that the profession attracts and retains nurses who are well suited to provide nursing care in these nontraditional settings. Between 2012 and 2022, job growth of registered nurses is expected to grow the most in non-hospital settings, with the largest growth expected in home healthcare (43% increase), followed by outpatient ambulatory care (40% increase), and long-term care (24% increase). Nursing jobs in the inpatient hospital setting are only expected to increase by 15% during this time period (Center for Health and Workforce Studies, 2014). Another source reported that the volume of outpatient services is expected to grow 17% over the next 5 years, whereas inpatient discharges are expected to decrease by 3% (Department of Health & Human Services, 2013).

This book focuses on describing 60 community-based, non-hospital careers in nursing. The various careers are organized according to population-focused care. Population-focused care is care that involves evaluating and treating the health needs of a population as a whole rather than individuals (Kulbok, Thatcher, Park, & Meszaros, 2012). In this book, these populations are organized by age categories, starting from newborns and progressing through older adults. This organization method coincides with the developmental stages of life, which is a concept that is part of most all nursing education programs, and familiar to nurses. The last section of the book includes nursing careers that are not specific to one of the aforementioned developmental stages, but instead focuses on a unique role within nursing and healthcare. Each of the 60 non-hospital nursing careers includes a basic description of the job, the educational preparation or skills that are required, typical work hours and settings, availability of specialty certifications associated with the job, and links to professional organizations and online resources for that specialty. The goal of this book is to inform practicing nurses and those who currently are or will be pursuing a career in nursing about the various non-hospital career options. This book is recommended to be used by nurse educators teaching nursing students about their practice options before they become licensed registered nurses.

Why Is This Book Needed?

Although there are a few books that focus on various careers in nursing, there are no books that focus exclusively on non-hospital careers in nursing. As mentioned before, there is an ongoing shift in our healthcare system from acute to community-based care settings that will require an expanded nursing workforce. This workforce should be diverse and prepared to care for a diverse population in nontraditional settings of care. This book provides information to students and others interested in the profession about their future options for careers in nursing, and to nurses who are already practicing in the profession with alternative nursing careers in non-hospital settings. It can be a useful resource to nurse educators who teach in academic nursing programs who could incorporate the various career options found in this book within their academic courses. This book would make a great additional resource that can be used alongside a community or public health nursing course.

Who Should Read This Book?

- Practicing nurses (novice to expert)
- Nursing students currently enrolled in a program
- Individuals interested in pursuing a career in nursing
- Academic nursing faculty and educators
- Nursing administrators and deans
- High school guidance counselors and advisors

What Makes This Book Different From Similar Books About Careers in Nursing?

This book focuses on only non-hospital nursing jobs, whereas similar books focus on all nursing specialties, most of which are in the hospital. An RN (registered nurse) license is the basic educational level requirement for most of the jobs discussed in this book. Although there are some non-hospital nursing jobs that require advanced practice education, the intent of this book is to focus on jobs that nurses with a basic undergraduate educational preparation in nursing can obtain, such as with an associate or baccalaureate degree. Books with a similar focus include content on all nursing careers, many of which do require advanced education at the master's or doctorate level. This book provides information about career options for nurses who cannot or do not want to pursue an advanced degree in nursing.

This book is uniquely organized according to care population age ranges/developmental stages (i.e., infants, children, adolescents/young adults, adults, and older adults). Lastly, several of the non-hospital nursing careers include a short excerpt from a nurse who is currently working in the field. This was designed to provide the reader with a real-life description of what it is like working in that specific non-hospital nursing role. The excerpts help highlight some of the details and benefits of that particular nursing job as described by a real-life nurse who is practicing in that role.

Origins of Nursing Outside the Hospital Setting

The first accounts of what we know as nursing care were recorded through early writings of physicians during Babylonian times (Joel, 2006). In these writings, physicians described various care and treatments that were given to the sick by some type of lay nurse that included diet, enemas, and bandaging (Joel, 2006). Prior to the 1800s, nurses were not formally trained or educated and learned their skills from what was passed down to them generation to generation. Most of the "nursing care" was informal and given at home by women family members or women affiliated with a religious order or congregation (Stanhope & Lancaster, 2014). The first "nurses" were often perceived in an unpleasant manner by the public as being incompetent, immoral, and drunk (Judd, Sitzman, & Davis, 2010). Women who came from good families and proper social upbringings were not thought to be fit to be nurses. Florence Nightingale was one of these women who led a revolution in changing this perception. Coming from a wealthy family, she went against her family's wishes and became a nurse. Among nurses, she is thought of as the first nurse and pioneer for nursing practice. She is also considered by some to be the first nurse researcher and nurse epidemiologist because she collected and tracked the mortality rates of the soldiers she cared for during the Crimean War (Stanhope & Lancaster, 2014). She began to examine whether some of the nursing interventions given to soldiers helped to improve their mortality rates. She determined that a good diet, cleanliness, and proper ventilation were critical in helping to improve outcomes for soldiers (Fee & Garafolo, 2010). This can be considered the first example of evidence-based practice as we know it today. All of these examples of the early accounts of nursing practice showed that nurses went where patients were (home, battlefield, etc.) to provide care. Non-hospital-based nursing was really the start of the profession of nursing as we know it today.

The profession of nursing began to evolve after the end of the American Civil War. There was a great increase in the building of hospitals, which also led to the development of the first formal training programs in nursing. This shift in where the sick were cared for—from the home to the hospital—changed the dynamic of both nursing care and how people died in the United States. Nurses, who previously cared for the sick at home, now worked in the hospital. Advancements in medical science and technology were occurring that further enabled the growth of hospitals all over the country. The start of what we know as traditional hospital-based nursing was born (Lowey, 2015). In the late 1800s and early 1900s, trained nurses had mainly two options for nursing jobs: work in private duty in homes or try to get a position working in a hospital, which was not easy to obtain during that time (Joel, 2006). Many nurses continued to provide private care for patients in their homes or went on to provide care for the public in general.

This time marked the period of industrialization in America, where millions of immigrants flocked to large cities in search of work. Overcrowding and poor sanitation precipitated the establishment of many public health initiatives. Although hospital-oriented nursing was rapidly growing, non-hospital nursing care did not disappear and started to flourish in the early 1900s. Nurses have always been there to provide care to individuals and families from all socioeconomic and geographic areas in non-hospital settings. The development of public or community health nursing as we know it today occurred in two very different geographies: urban and rural. Settlement houses or neighborhood centers were established in urban areas as places that offered healthcare and social welfare programs for the public. Lillian Wald and Mary Brewster were two nurses that started making home visits to the poor living in New York's Lower East Side. This led to the development of the Henry Street Settlement, which later progressed into the Visiting Nurse Service of America (Stanhope & Lancaster, 2014). Nearly 50,000 nursing visits were made to over 5,000 patients in New York City. Similar urban public health initiatives led by nurses were occurring in other areas of the United States, such as in Boston and Chicago.

School nursing began its origins during this time and was developed as an extension of home visiting in New York City. In the early 1900s, it was not uncommon for one-fifth of children to be absent from school on any given day (Stanhope & Lancaster, 2014). Thousands of students were sent home from school regularly for any type of illness, even if small. Nurses would visit and treat students at home for scabies, lice, ringworm, and other dermatological ailments that often resulted from tenement living (Judd et al., 2010). Other students were absent due to lack of proper food or clothing or having to take care of younger siblings at home while parents engaged in factory work (Stanhope & Lancaster, 2014). These visiting nurses cared about these often socially-based issues that affected the health of the schoolchildren and were great advocates for educating parents and promoting health during this time period. Through this, school nursing was formally established.

Industrial nursing, which was nursing care that developed from home visiting, later progressed into what we know today as occupational health nursing. In the late 1800s, Betty Moulder—who provided health services to a group of coal miners in Pennsylvania—was the first documented industrial or occupational health nurse (Joel, 2006). She was followed by Ada Mayo Stewart, who began working with employees of the Vermont Marble Company in Proctor, Vermont. Nurses were being hired to provide healthcare services for employees in other businesses, such as department stores and manufacturing operations (Stanhope & Lancaster, 2014). It wasn't until 1958 that the term *occupational health nurse* was adopted through the American Nurses Association (Joel, 2006).

The Frontier Nursing Service was the first rural healthcare system in America, and it was established by a nurse. Mary Breckinridge established the Frontier Nursing Service in Kentucky in the mid 1920s after recognition of a great need for maternity care in the region (Judd et al., 2010). Women were not getting adequate prenatal or postnatal care, and that greatly affected the health of both mothers and infants. Breckinridge and several other nurses made home visits to rural residents in Appalachia either on horseback or foot. Their care was often the only care pregnant women and new mothers would receive. Nursing midwifery, mother-baby home care nursing, and rural nursing resulted from the work of Breckinridge and others with the Frontier Nursing Service.

Conclusion

Public health, home care, school, occupational health, and rural nursing are only a few of the many types of non-hospital nursing careers that are available for nurses. Each of these settings is flourishing and being practiced by thousands of nurses all over the country. Over the years, other non-hospital nursing careers have emerged as viable practice areas for nurses who want to work with special populations and provide different types of nursing care to patients in all developmental stages of life, afflicted by both acute and chronic conditions, in every geographic corner of the country. Some of these more specialized and perhaps less well-known careers are directly derived from the original non-hospital careers that have been described, while others developed as a result to meet a specific need in our expanding healthcare system. Several of the 60 non-hospital careers discussed in this book have a specialty board certification that nurses can acquire to become recognized as an expert in that particular field. In addition to the well-known professional associations for nurses, such as the Honor Society of Nursing, Sigma Theta Tau International and the American Nurses Association, there are numerous other professional organizations that are associated with the nursing specialties that are identified in this book. If available, both specialty certifications and professional organizations are listed with each non-hospital nursing career.

Nurses who practice outside of the hospital often take on various roles and responsibilities to deliver comprehensive healthcare to their patients. Some of the most common roles can include caregiver, educator, change agent, advocate, leader, case manager, community advocate, public policy developer, program planner, and researcher. The level of care that nurses provide can differ between each type of non-hospital nursing job. For example, a nurse who works as a mother-baby home care nurse will likely be most engaged as a caregiver and educator, whereas a nurse who works in a public health domain may be more involved with planning programs and developing health policies. The specific focus of care of the "patient" also differs with each type of non-hospital nursing job. The focus might be one person, the patient, or it might be an entire family unit. Or the focus may be even broader and take on larger groups of people, such as entire communities or populations of people.

Regardless of the focus, the progression of nursing as profession has grown substantially over the past several decades. Nurses collaborate with other healthcare disciplines, are involved in policy-making initiatives, conduct and/or evaluate and incorporate research into their practice settings, and have developed a strong voice in the healthcare system. The growth in our profession can be attributed to many factors; however, the care and services that nurses provide in nontraditional care settings have greatly contributed to this growth. As with the first nurses who had the drive to help those less fortunate in the overcrowded tenements in New York City to those nurses that rode endless hours on horseback to help women and children in Appalachia, nurses have always been there to help those in need.

References

Center for Health Care Workforce Studies. (May 2014). Health care employment projections: An analysis of bureau labor statistics, settings and occupational projections, 2012–2022. Retrieved from http://chws.albany.edu/archive/uploads/2014/08/blsproj2014.pdf

Department of Health & Human Services. (April 2013). The U.S. nursing workforce: Trends in supply and education. Retrieved from http://bhpr.hrsa.gov/healthworkforce/reports/nursingworkforce/nursingworkforcefullreport.pdf

Fee, E., & Garofalo, M. E. (2010). Florence Nightingale and the Crimean War. *American Journal of Public Health, 100*(9), 1591.

Institute of Medicine of the National Academies Committee on the Robert Wood Johnson Foundation Initiative on the Future of Nursing. (2008). *The future of nursing: Leading change, advancing health.* Retrieved from http://www.ic4n.org/wp-content/uploads/2012/01/Future-of-Nursing-Leading-Change-Advancing-Health.pdf

Joel, L. A. (2006). *The nursing experience: Trends, challenges, and transitions* (5th ed.). New York, NY: McGraw-Hill.

Judd, D., Sitzman, K., & Davis, G. M. (2010). *A history of American nursing: Trends and eras.* Sudbury, MA: Jones & Bartlett.

Kulbok, P. A., Thatcher, E., Park, E., & Meszaros, P. S. (2012). Evolving public health nursing roles: Focus on community participatory health promotion and prevention. *The Online Journal of Issues in Nursing, 17*(2). Retrieved from http://nursingworld.org/MainMenuCategories/ANAMarketplace/ANAPeriodicals/OJIN/TableofContents/Vol-17-2012/No2-May-2012/Evolving-Public-Health-Nursing-Roles.html

Lowey, S. E. (2015). *Nursing care at the end of life: What every clinician should know*. Geneseo, NY: SUNY Open Textbooks.

Stanhope, M., & Lancaster, J. (2014). *Foundations of nursing in the community: Community oriented practice* (4th ed.). St. Louis, MO: Mosby Elsevier.

PART 1

NEWBORNS AND INFANTS

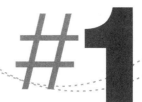

CHILDBIRTH EDUCATOR

Job Description

Childbirth education is an important component of prenatal care. The role of a childbirth educator is to provide educational information about various components of childbirth, including pregnancy, labor and delivery, postpartum care, and breastfeeding. The childbirth educator nurse can develop, implement, and evaluate education classes that can be used with a diverse population of expectant families. They can provide resources, information, and support for expectant mothers.

Typical Work Hours and Setting

Childbirth educators can be employed in a variety of inpatient and outpatient settings, including physician and obstetric offices, community health centers, and home healthcare agencies. They can implement education classes in a facility and/or in the home setting. Work hours vary, but childbirth educators may often need to work evening and weekend hours to accommodate the work schedule for expectant parents.

Education and Training Requirements

- Must be currently licensed as an RN in the United States.
- Most often requires experience working with expectant mothers in labor and delivery.
- Must possess good interpersonal and communication skills.
- Education experience is recommended.
- Should be free of physical restrictions that can impede the ability to get down on the floor for demonstration during classes.

Specialty Certification

Nurses can become nationally certified as a Childbirth Educator through the International Childbirth Education Association's Professional Childbirth Educator (PCBE) Certification Program or through the Prepared Childbirth Educators, Inc. Childbirth Educator Certification Examination. Each organization has its own criteria, but generally, nurses need to have experience in the role of a Childbirth Educator and may be required to have a number of continuing education contact hours to sit for the exam.

Professional Organizations and Online Resources

The International Childbirth Education Association: http://icea.org/

Childbirth and Postpartum Professional Association: http://www.cappa.net/

Prepared Childbirth Educators, Inc: https://www.childbirtheducation.org/

Childbirth Professionals International: http://thechildbirthprofession.com/

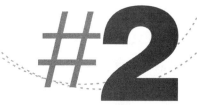

GENETICS NURSE

Job Description

Genetics nurses, otherwise known as *genetics clinical nurses,* are registered nurses with special training in genetics. They care for patients who have or are at risk to develop diseases that have a genetic component, such as heart disease, diabetes, and Alzheimer's. They can also work with patients who have been born with hereditary genetic defects or disorders. Genetics clinical nurses provide nursing assessment and formulate a plan of care with a focus on genetic factors. This includes taking a detailed family history, providing education about genetic disorders, and providing support to patients and families.

Typical Work Hours and Setting

Genetics clinical nurses can be employed in a variety of inpatient and outpatient settings, including physician offices, genetics clinics, prenatal and reproductive centers, research centers, and the biotechnology and insurance industries. They can implement education classes in a facility and/or in the home setting. Work hours vary, but genetics nurses may often need to work evening and weekend hours to accommodate the work schedule for expectant parents.

Education and Training Requirements

- Must be currently licensed as an RN in the United States.
- Must have a baccalaureate degree in nursing.
- Must possess good interpersonal, listening, and communication skills.
- Must possess a good level of maturity and sensitivity to patient concerns.

Specialty Certification

Until recently, nurses were able to become certified as a Genetics Clinical Nurse (GCN) through the Genetic Nurses Credentialing Commission. Nurses who currently possess this former certification can renew through the American Nurses Credentialing Center, but new applicants are no longer being accepted for this exam. Nurses who want to become certified in genetics now must have graduate level education and can sit for the Advanced Genetics Nursing Exam and become board certified as an AGN-BC.

Professional Organizations and Online Resources

International Society of Nurses in Genetics: http://www.isong.org/

Genomic Careers: https://www.genome.gov/genomiccareers/career.cfm?id=22

National Society of Genetics Counselors: http://www.nsgc.org/

American Board of Genetic Counseling: http://www.abgc.net/ABGC/AmericanBoardofGeneticCounselors.asp

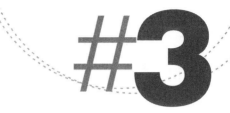

LACTATION CONSULTANT

Job Description

Lactation consultants work in the area of women's health and focus their care on new mothers who are breastfeeding. They assess both the mother and infant, including history, physical examination, and feeding observation. They can help educate the mother on feeding and troubleshoot feeding-related problems. Lactation consultants can also provide education and information that would benefit new mothers, including nutrition and exercise. They also provide good support and encouragement.

Typical Work Hours and Setting

Lactation consultants can be employed in a variety of inpatient and outpatient settings, including hospitals, birthing centers, obstetric offices, home healthcare agencies, and as private consultants. They can facilitate breastfeeding classes in a facility and/or in the clinic setting. Work hours vary, but lactation consultants may often need to work evening and weekend hours to accommodate the work schedule for new mothers.

Education and Training Requirements

- Must be currently licensed as an RN in the United States.
- Most often requires experience working with new mothers in labor and delivery and/or neonatal nursing.
- Should have a good knowledge of women's health, lactation, and breastfeeding.
- Must possess good interpersonal and communication skills.

Specialty Certification

Nurses can become certified as an International Board Certified Lactation Consultant (IBCLC) through the International Board of Lactation Consultant Examiners. To be eligible, nurses must demonstrate they have 1,000 hours of clinical practice in lactation and breastfeeding care that was obtained within the 5 years immediately prior to applying for the exam. This exam also requires nurses to have had coursework in specific health science subjects, lactation, and breastfeeding, and also clinical experience working with new mothers.

Professional Organizations and Online Resources

United States Lactation Consultant Association: https://uslca.org/

International Lactation Consultant Association: http://www.ilca.org/home

International Board of Lactation Consultant Examiners: http://iblce.org/

Lactation Education Resources: https://www.lactationtraining.com/our-courses/online-courses/lactation-consultant-training-program

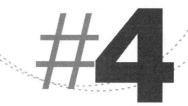

MATERNAL-CHILD HEALTH NURSE

Job Description

Maternal-child health nurses provide care to families by supporting the development of children from birth until school age and their parents. In addition to monitoring the health of the child, they also focus on the health of the parent(s) and identify health-related or developmental issues early. Part of this role includes assessment of the interaction between child and parent(s) and development of a plan of care that includes fostering the mother-child and/ or father-child relationship. The maternal-child health nurse also provides relevant education and information to promote healthy behaviors and provides support for parents.

Typical Work Hours and Setting

Maternal-child health nurses can be employed in a variety of inpatient and outpatient settings, including physician, obstetric, and pediatric offices; community health centers; and public health and home healthcare agencies. They often work in public or home health agencies and make home visits to families with new infants. Work hours vary, but maternal-child health nurses may often need to work evening and weekend hours to accommodate the work schedule for families.

Education and Training Requirements

- Must be currently licensed as an RN in the United States.
- Experience working with families in women's health; maternity or pediatrics is preferred.
- Prior home care experience is beneficial (if working in home healthcare).
- Must possess good interpersonal, listening, and communication skills.
- Should have a good understanding of the availability of local resources for families.

Specialty Certification

There is currently no certification exam specifically for maternal-child nursing at the RN level. However, nurses can sit for the pediatric, ambulatory care, or nursing case management certification exam through the American Nurses Credentialing Center.

Professional Organizations and Online Resources

Childbirth and Postpartum Professional Association: http://www.cappa.net/

Prepared Childbirth Educators, Inc: https://www.childbirtheducation.org/

Childbirth Professionals International: http://thechildbirthprofession.com/

Maternal-Child Health Nurse Leadership Academy: http://www.nursingsociety.org/learn-grow/leadership-institute/maternal-child-health-nurse-leadership-academy

American Nurses Credentialing Center: http://www.nursecredentialing.org/certification.aspx

PART **2**

CHILDREN, ADOLESCENTS, AND YOUNG ADULTS

5

CAMP NURSE

Job Description

Camp nurses provide medical care to individuals of all ages who are attending a camp or retreat. Most often, camp nurses work with the pediatric population since tens of thousands of children have a camp experience each year. They can assess and treat both acute and chronic conditions of the campers and staff in the camp environment. This often includes injuries and conditions resulting from camping such as bug bites or stings, dermatological issues related to the outdoor environment such as reactions to poison ivy, sprains, and other minor injuries and burns. Camp nurses should possess the ability to respond to emergent situations, if needed. Camp nurses can provide basic education about hygiene, first aid, food, and camping safety.

Typical Work Hours and Setting

Although camp nursing is most often thought of as a seasonal position, full-time camp nurse jobs are available. The seasonal position is most often available through the summer months and is outdoors. Benefits to camp nurses include the provision of free room and board during employment at the camp.

Education and Training Requirements

- Must be currently licensed as an RN in the United States.
- Must have basic CPR for the healthcare professional certification.
- Advanced life support (ALS) certification is a plus.
- Must possess good interpersonal and communication skills.
- Experience working with children is highly recommended.
- Should be free of physical restrictions that can impede ability to be in an outdoor setting.

Specialty Certification

Although there currently is no national certification available for camp nurses through the American Nurses Credentialing Center, nurses are able to obtain a certificate in camp nursing through Bemidji State University. The camp nursing certificate was developed and endorsed by both the Association of Camp Nurses and the American Camp Association.

Professional Organizations and Online Resources

Association of Camp Nurses:
http://www.acn.org/

American Camp Association:
http://www.acacamps.org/

Camp Nurse Jobs.com:
http://www.campnursejobs.com/

Bemidji State University Camp Nursing Certificate:
http://www.bemidjistate.edu/academics/graduate-studies/programs/camp-nursing/

6

CHILD PSYCHIATRIC/ MENTAL HEALTH NURSE

Job Description

The focus of a child psychiatric/mental health nurse is on promotion of optimal mental health, assessment of mental health status, implementing interventions to regain or improve patients' coping abilities, and preventing further mental health disability. Child mental health nurses help to foster a therapeutic environment, implement and evaluate psychobiological interventions, and educate patients and families about mental healthcare. Nurses may also assist with crisis intervention, mental health counseling, and case management for pediatric and adolescent patients.

Typical Work Hours and Setting

Child psychiatric/mental health nurses can be employed in a variety of inpatient and outpatient settings, including outpatient psychiatric facilities and clinics, psychiatrist and primary care physician offices, child protective or welfare agencies, foster care services, and juvenile justice and other child-focused community or public health agencies. Work hours vary according to the specific agency of employment.

Education and Training Requirements

- Must be currently licensed as an RN in the United States.
- Should have experience working with pediatric and/or psychiatric patient population.
- Must possess excellent interpersonal, listening, and communication skills.
- Must be able to foster a therapeutic and trustworthy relationship with patients and families.

Specialty Certification

Nurses can become board certified as a Psychiatric-Mental Health Nurse through the American Nurses Credentialing Center. This certification focuses on mental health in both the child and adult populations. Nurses who are interested in pursuing focused specialty certification in child/adolescent psychiatric mental health must do so at the clinical nurse specialist level, which requires a master's degree.

Professional Organizations and Online Resources

American Psychiatric Nurses Association: http://www.apna.org/

American Academy of Child & Adolescent Psychiatry: http://www.aacap.org/

International Society of Psychiatric-Mental Health Nurses: http://www.ispn-psych.org/

American Nurses Credentialing Center: http://www.nursecredentialing.org/certification.aspx

Psychiatric Nursing.com: http://www.psychiatricnursing.com/home

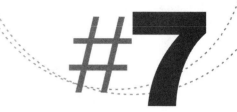

COLLEGE HEALTH CENTER NURSE

Job Description

College health center nurses work on college and university campuses and are involved in the care of young adult college students. Using the nursing process, college health nurses provide individualized care for this population. This includes assessment of physical, psychosocial, emotional, and environmental stressors for the student. They act as a resource to the college and provide education about health promotion and disease prevention to students, faculty, and staff. The college health nurse participates in college-wide health fairs and events, organizes and promotes influenza education and clinics, coordinates mandatory screenings for international students, and educates students about risky behaviors and topics of concern to the college student population.

Typical Work Hours and Setting

Nurses who work in college health centers typically work when school is in session and may have reduced hours during summer and/or winter breaks. Nurses may work in another per diem position when the college is closed. Nurses work in the health center but may provide health screenings and education in other locations across the campus and in the community at large.

Education and Training Requirements

- Must be currently licensed as an RN in the United States.
- Must have basic life support (BLS) and/or CPR certification.
- Should possess knowledge of college health requirements such as vaccinations.
- Must possess good interpersonal, listening, and communication skills.
- Should be prepared to work with students from diverse backgrounds and cultures.

Specialty Certification

The board certification for College Health Nurse through the American Nurses Credentialing Center is no longer being offered. Nurses who work in college health may become certified in ambulatory care through the American Nurses Credentialing Center.

Professional Organizations and Online Resources

American College Health Association:
http://www.acha.org/

American Nurses Association:
http://www.nursingworld.org/

American Nurses Credentialing Center:
http://www.nursecredentialing.org/certification

Sigma Theta Tau International Honor Society of Nursing:
http://www.nursingsociety.org/

career highlight

Staff Nurse at the Student Health Center

Darlene Zeliff, BSN, RN

Q: What led you to your current career in nursing?

A: Before coming to the college, I had worked 12-hour shifts in a small emergency department for about 20 years. I had thought that this would be a much easier job. It isn't "easier," but it is different. We have been rotating Saturday hours, which is better than whole weekends or 12-hour shifts. The Student Health Center flows at a steady pace and sometimes can get quite busy. It is similar to an urgent care/primary care center, and we see patients with acute respiratory illnesses, gynecological concerns, etc.

Q: What are your typical job duties and responsibilities?

A: Typically I triage patients to be seen and evaluated by an NP (nurse practitioner). I obtain their vital signs, medical/social/family history, and medication history. I anticipate the needs of the NP and assist by obtaining the needed samples such as urine to test for pregnancy and/or urinary tract infections, throat cultures to test for strep, etc. I start intravenous medications (IVs) and give injections under the direction of the NP. I am also able to discharge some patients myself if they have uncomplicated problems or after discussion with the NP. We also have "nurse appointments" for STD screenings. I also perform phlebotomy as needed.

Q: Is there any special training or education required for your job?

A: Since I began working at the health center, I have received various training and learned different responsibilities that I never performed while working at the hospital. I am able to work closely with the international college student population, particularly in regard to screening for tuberculosis (TB). I have learned so much about TB, the high-risk countries from which students come that have higher incidence of TB, and the various screenings used for TB. At the beginning of every semester, I speak to the new international students to discuss the services that the health center has to offer. It is fun to see their recognition when they come to the health center and seek me out as a resource. I am also in charge of Vaccines for Children, another area that I had to learn for this position. Since college students have to show proof of mandatory vaccinations required by law and many of our students travel abroad, I have to be educated on this topic for my role. I have learned about the state-wide program for Vaccines for Children. I am also in charge of mandatory education for the staff at the health center. This includes the development of educational materials and oversight of our annual in-service. Additionally, I am also often in the role as a nurse preceptor and provide mentorship of the nursing students that host each semester.

Q: What is the best part of your job?

A: The patients in this job, as in the emergency department, are always changing. I enjoy the variety of patients and I like the one-on-one interaction with college students. I also like that we often see the same patients (such as in primary care), and we can see how they are improving and learning to care for themselves. I enjoy the rapport I have with the students and the close working relationships I have with the providers.

Q: What is the least favorite part of your job?

A: Politics. I am sure that occurs in any nursing job that is out there.

Q: What advice would you give to those interested in pursuing a career in your nursing field?

A: I have been in my current position for almost 8 years, and there have been many changes over this time. Changes to the nursing positions and scheduling and the addition of the electronic medical record have changed the work environment. Our administration is very forward-thinking, and that requires change. I would tell people interested in this field to be flexible. Some changes are difficult, but other changes can make life and the nursing role easier and more organized. No matter what nursing career you are in, times change and nurses need to be prepared for it.

Q: Anything important that you would like nurses to know about your nursing job?

A: I love nursing as a profession in general and any kind of nursing. I feel this job is usually less stressful, so hopefully I am kind to the patients I see here. Hopefully this runs over into my per diem job and I am not exhausted and have more patience there. I appreciate the flexibility that nursing has to offer. I have worked many different hours, days, and locations in my 35+ years as a nurse. Nursing has the ability to be flexible in whatever stage of life I am in.

#8

DEVELOPMENTAL DISABILITIES NURSE

Job Description

Developmental disabilities nurses, also known as *special needs nurses,* work with patients who have a physical or mental developmental disability. Nurses provide and facilitate services and care for persons with intellectual or developmental disabilities in order to promote optimal functioning and independence and increase quality of life. Developmental disabilities nurses can provide skilled nursing care, such as assisting patients with bathing, feeding, and toileting; work in the capacity of a case manager and coordinate care and services for patients; act as a patient advocate; and offer education and information to patients with developmental disabilities and their families.

Typical Work Hours and Setting

Nurses who work with developmentally disabled persons can work in various settings, including schools, primary care, group homes, and community-based agencies. They can provide care to developmentally disabled persons who are residing in their home or are at their school or work setting. Nurses who work in group home settings may have evening, nighttime, and/or weekend hours and may also be required to offer on-call support with their position. They may additionally be required to accompany their patients for travel outside the facility on community outings.

Education and Training Requirements

- Must be currently licensed as an RN in the United States.
- Must possess good interpersonal, listening, and communication skills.
- Should exhibit patience and compassion for the developmentally disabled population.

Specialty Certification

The registered nurse Certification in Developmental Disabilities Nursing (CDDN) is the certification that nurses can acquire through the Developmental Disabilities Nurses Association. To qualify, nurses must meet the practice requirement, which is a minimum of 4,000 hours of active practice in the care of persons with developmental disabilities in the past 5 years.

Professional Organizations and Online Resources

Developmental Disabilities Nurses Association: https://ddna.org/

American Association on Intellectual and Developmental Disabilities: https://aaidd.org/

Association of Professional Developmental Disabilities Administrators: http://www.apdda.org/

9

DOMESTIC VIOLENCE NURSE

Job Description

Domestic violence nurses work in the sub-specialty of forensics nursing and care for patients who are or have been the victim of some type of violence. Most often, nurses may work with women and children who have been victims of domestic violence, but can also work with the elderly population in elder abuse type of violence cases. These nurses provide assessment and care for those affected by domestic violence and are also critical in the identification and documentation of these cases. Domestic violence nurses are often called to legal proceedings to provide expert testimony and can also be sought out as consultants in these legal cases. Nurses who work with victims of domestic violence act as advocates and help to educate the public about the importance of early recognition and intervention of victims of violence.

Typical Work Hours and Setting

Domestic violence nurses can work in a variety of settings, including the emergency department, outpatient clinics, community-based advocacy centers, and women's health and senior health networks. Work hours vary but may include working evening, night, weekend, and on-call hours.

Education and Training Requirements

- Must be currently licensed as an RN in the United States.
- Should have excellent assessment and documentation skills.
- Must possess good interpersonal, listening, and communication skills.
- Must provide sensitivity and confidentiality toward patients.

Specialty Certification

There are two certification options for nurses who work in domestic violence nursing positions. The first is the Sexual Assault Nurse Examiner (SANE) certification through the International Association of Forensic Nurses. To qualify, nurses must have a minimum of 2 years of experience working in an area where they have practiced advanced physical assessment skills, such as emergency or critical care. Then they must receive specialized SANE education, which includes both classroom and clinical components. The American Nurses Credentialing Center also offers Certification in Advanced Forensic Nursing, but this requires graduate level education.

Professional Organizations and Online Resources

International Association of Forensic Nurses: http://www.forensicnurses.org/

American Nurses Credentialing Center: http://www.nursecredentialing.org/certification

National Resource Center on Domestic Violence: http://www.nrcdv.org/dvrn/

National Center on Domestic Violence, Trauma & Mental Health: http://www.nationalcenterdvtraumamh.org/

#10

PEDIATRIC HOME CARE NURSE

Job Description

Pediatric home care nurses make home visits to provide skilled nursing care to children and their families. They work with newborns, infants, toddlers and preschoolers, school-aged children, and adolescents who have an illness or injury that requires nursing care in the home. Nurses can provide care either for a short-term basis for an acute condition or long term for chronic medical care. Pediatric home care nurses use the nursing process to provide individualized care for pediatric patients to promote healing, restore optimal functioning, facilitate developmental growth, and improve quality of life for the patient and family.

Typical Work Hours and Setting

Pediatric home care nurses can work for certified home health agencies, public health departments, or other pediatric community or advocacy agencies that offer home visiting services. Work hours vary and may include evening, weekend, and on-call hours. Nurses travel various distances to make visits to patients' homes. Length of home visits may vary according to need. Nurses often need to coordinate care between the home and pediatric provider to facilitate necessary interventions.

Education and Training Requirements

- Must be currently licensed as an RN in the United States.
- Most often requires experience working in the acute care setting with children.
- Must possess good interpersonal, listening, communication, and organizational skills.
- Home care experience is preferred.

Specialty Certification

Although there is no specific certification exam for pediatric home care nurses, nurses can become nationally certified in pediatric or public health nursing, depending on the primary focus of their position. Both the American Nurses Credentialing Center and the Pediatric Nursing Certification Board offer certification examinations.

Professional Organizations and Online Resources

Pediatric Nursing Certification Board: https://www.pncb.org/ptistore/control/exams/pn/index

Institute of Pediatric Nursing: http://www.ipedsnursing.org/ptisite/control/index

National Association of Pediatric Nurse Practitioners: https://www.napnap.org/

American Academy of Pediatrics: https://www.aap.org/

#11

PEDIATRIC PALLIATIVE CARE NURSE

Job Description

Pediatric palliative care nursing is a fairly new sub-specialty that bridges pediatric and hospice/palliative nursing. The pediatric palliative care nurse provides care to children and adolescents who have been diagnosed with a life-threatening illness. Using a palliative philosophy of care, nursing assessments and interventions are focused on providing comfort and improving quality of life for patients and families. Pediatric palliative care nurses usually work as part of a team that includes other healthcare workers such as doctors, social workers, and chaplains. Pediatric patients are cared for holistically by focusing on physical, psychological, social, and spiritual aspects of care at the developmental stage they are in.

Typical Work Hours and Setting

Childbirth educators can be employed in a variety of inpatient and outpatient settings, including pediatric specialist physician offices, inpatient hospital pediatric or palliative care services, pediatric ambulatory and cancer care centers, and home healthcare agencies.

Education and Training Requirements

- Must be currently licensed as an RN in the United States.
- Nurses should have experience working with children who have serious illnesses or injuries such as in the pediatric intensive care unit, pediatric emergency department, pediatric oncology/hematology, and neonatal intensive care unit.
- Must possess good interpersonal, listening, and communication skills.
- Should be able to give sensitive and compassionate care to children with serious illnesses and their families.

Specialty Certification

Nurses can become nationally certified as a Certified Hospice & Palliative Pediatric Nurse (CHPPN) through the Hospice & Palliative Credentialing Center. To be eligible, nurses have to have a minimum of 500 hours in the past year in pediatric palliative care. Nurses can also receive specialty training in pediatric palliative care through the End of Life Nursing Education Consortium (ELNEC). ELNEC offers several training workshops annually throughout the country.

Professional Organizations and Online Resources

The Initiative for Pediatric Palliative Care: http://www.ippcweb.org/

National Hospice and Palliative Care Organization: http://www.nhpco.org/pediatric

Hospice & Palliative Credentialing Center: http://hpcc.advancingexpertcare.org/competence/rn-peds-chppn/

End of Life Nursing Education Consortium: http://www.aacn.nche.edu/elnec/about/pediatric-palliative-care

12

SCHOOL NURSE

Job Description

School nurses have a vital role in the school community to provide expertise and oversight for the provision of school health services and the promotion of health education. Using the nursing process, the school nurse provides healthcare to students and staff who become ill or injured, conducts mandatory health screenings, and helps to coordinate care between the home healthcare provider and school. School nurses also must be knowledgeable about and compliant with maintaining students' immunization documentation. They are also often involved in the tracking of student attendance and absences from the school. School nurses may also provide and coordinate health education in the school and teach students and staff about various ways to promote healthy behaviors.

Typical Work Hours and Setting

School nurses typically work during the months when school is in session and have holiday and summer breaks off from their position. School nurses may also need to accompany students on school outings, field trips, and after-school sporting events. Some school nurses may work in clinical practice over summer break. In addition to the clinical responsibilities, many school nurses are responsible for administrative work related to documentation and record-keeping of health records.

Education and Training Requirements

- Must be currently licensed as an RN in the United States.
- Most often requires prior experience working with children in the acute care setting.
- Must possess good interpersonal, listening, and communication skills with children.
- Education experience is recommended for school nurses involved in health education programming.

Specialty Certification

The American Nurses Credentialing Center no longer offers the school nurse certification exam. Nurses who want to obtain specialty certification as a school nurse can go through the National Board for Certification of School Nurses. To be eligible, nurses must meet the clinical practice requirements, which include a minimum of 1,000 hours of school nursing worked during the past 3 years. The school nurse board certification is good for 5 years, at which time nurses have the option to recertify.

Professional Organizations and Online Resources

National Association of School Nurses: http://www.nasn.org/

American School Health Association: http://www.ashaweb.org/

National Board for Certification of School Nurses: http://www.nbcsn.org/

School Nurse.com: http://www.schoolnurse.com/public/department42.cfm

career highlight

School Nurse/Health Coordinator

Jennifer K. Manley, BS, RN

Q: What led you to your current career in nursing?

A: My calling to be in the health profession started many years before this. I enjoyed taking care of my great-grandmother with all her health needs, and then I was a candy striper volunteering to help staff and patients in need. These experiences aided in my decision to enter the health profession. During my junior year of high school I began my nursing career, studying to be a nurse. Through perseverance of many obstacles in life, I was able to obtain my nursing degree and work myself up the professional ladder gaining an array of experience in a broad range of specialties in nursing, along with transitioning from the role of an LPN to that of a pediatric-centered registered nurse with a 4-year degree.

Q: What are your typical job duties and responsibilities?

A:
- Management of health appraisals/sports qualification
- NYS (New York State) mandated health screenings
- Immunization monitoring
- Survey and state reporting
- Medication administration
- Provision of first aid and nursing care
- Communicate disease management
- Blood-borne pathogen monitoring and training
- Allergy tracking and monitoring
- Development of healthcare plans for high-risk medical conditions
- In-services and to staff for high-risk medical conditions
- Collaboration with staff, parents, and administrators
- Assistance with attendance
- School committee involvements
- Promotion and education of health, wellness, and safety for the students and staff
- Evidence-based continuing education

Q: Is there any special training or education required for your job?

A: To be a school nurse there is no additional training required. Having a strong clinical experience in hospital-based nursing with a specialty in pediatrics is important. Other attributes that are beneficial to the public health/ambulatory care setting of school nursing are leadership skills, self-motivated team player, multi-tasking, prioritization, and able to gain a rapport with students and families.

Q: What is the best part of your job?

A: The best part of my job is being able to make a difference in the lives of every student, staff, and family that I care for!

Q: What is the least favorite part of your job?

A: Vomit! I have no others; I totally love and enjoy what I do. I look forward to coming to work every day!

Q: What advice would you give to those interested in pursuing a career in your nursing field?

A: As I examine the past 24 years of my nursing career, I am able to reflect on my experiences, personal accomplishments, and knowledge. I have learned that by maintaining a positive, dedicated, and nonjudgmental approach to my passion of nursing in the healthcare field, you can accomplish goals, develop and maintain lifelong professional friendships, along with connections to outside resources.

Q: Anything important that you would like nurses to know about your nursing job?

A: Knowledge of NYS educational laws, guidelines, and evidence-based nursing practice is very important in the role of a school nurse. Also having the skills to manage time, prioritizing tasks using the nursing process, and exercising sound judgment required to improve the quality of the healthcare within the educational setting for students, their families, staff, and administrators.

PART 3

ADULTS

#13

AMBULATORY CARE NURSE

Job Description

Ambulatory care nursing is a broad specialty of nursing practice that takes place outside of the inpatient hospital setting. Ambulatory care nurses provide care across the developmental life span of patients, families, communities, and populations in a variety of care settings. Although many nurses provide face-to-face nursing care to patients, some ambulatory care settings offer care through telecommunications such as telephone triage and telemedicine. Nurses who work in ambulatory care must possess excellent clinical reasoning skills and be able to practice autonomously through interdisciplinary collaborative relationships.

Typical Work Hours and Setting

Ambulatory care nurses can work in a variety of outpatient settings, including hospital-based outpatient clinics, ambulatory surgery and diagnostic medical procedures centers, telemedicine or telehealth offices, managed care organizations, freestanding independent or community centers, and Department of Veterans Affairs clinics. Work hours vary, but ambulatory care nurses often need to work evening, weekend, and on-call hours.

Education and Training Requirements

- Must be currently licensed as an RN in the United States.
- Most often requires prior inpatient acute care experience.
- Must possess good interpersonal, listening, and communication skills.
- Should possess good knowledge and competence in cultural diversity.

Specialty Certification

Nurses can become nationally certified in ambulatory care and receive the RN-BC designation through the American Nurses Credentialing Center. To be eligible, nurses must have been in practice as a registered nurse for a minimum of 2 years full time, have worked 2,000 hours in ambulatory care and/or telehealth nursing, and have completed 30 hours of continuing education in ambulatory care or telehealth.

Professional Organizations and Online Resources

American Academy of Ambulatory Care Nursing: https://www.aaacn.org/

American Nurses Credentialing Center: http://www.nursecredentialing.org/certification

Ambulatory Surgery Center Association: http://www.ascassociation.org/home

Accreditation Association for Ambulatory Health Care, Inc: http://www.aaahc.org/

#14

CARDIAC CATHETERIZATION NURSE

Job Description

Cardiac catheterization nurses specialize in cardiac care and care for patients who are undergoing a cardiac catheterization procedure. Nurses provide care for patients before, during, and after the procedure. The nurse assesses the patient's vital signs, obtains a health history, and prepares the patient for the procedure. After the procedure, the nurse monitors the patient and provides teaching and patient discharge instructions.

Typical Work Hours and Setting

Cardiac catheterization nurses can work in cardiac catheterization labs located most often in inpatient or ambulatory cardiac specialty care settings. Work hours are typically daytime, but some on-call or off shifts may be required to meet the needs of patients who require emergency catheterization.

Education and Training Requirements

- Must be currently licensed as an RN in the United States.
- Most often requires 2 to 3 years of acute cardiac nursing care.
- Must possess both basic and advanced cardiac life support certification.
- Should have excellent cardiopulmonary assessment skills.

Specialty Certification

Nurses can become nationally board certified as a Cardiac Vascular Nurse through the American Nurses Credentialing Center. To be eligible for the exam, nurses should have a minimum of 2,000 hours working as a registered nurse in a cardiac vascular setting during the last 3 years. Additionally, nurses must have completed at least 30 hours of continuing education in cardiac vascular nursing within the last 3 years. Nurses can also receive specialty certification through the American Association of Critical-Care Nurses in the subspecialties of cardiac surgery or cardiac medicine.

Professional Organizations and Online Resources

American Nurses Credentialing Center: http://www.nursecredentialing.org/certification

American Association of Critical-Care Nurses: http://www.aacn.org/

American Association of Heart Failure Nurses: http://www.aahfn.org/

American Heart Association: http://www.heart.org/HEARTORG/

#15

CERTIFIED ADDICTIONS REGISTERED NURSE

Job Description

An addictions nurse, also known in some states as an *addictions counselor,* provides nursing care to patients with various addictions. This can include patients who are dependent on substances such as nicotine, alcohol, and drugs. Patients with compulsive type behaviors may also be seen, such as those with addictions to food or gambling. Nurses assist patients with their recovery process, including management of pain, education about their addiction, implementing interventions for treatment, participating or leading individual or group counseling sessions, and providing support for patients and families undergoing addiction issues.

Typical Work Hours and Setting

Certified addictions registered nurses can be employed in a variety of inpatient and outpatient settings, including physician and psychiatry offices, mental health centers, substance abuse rehabilitation facilities, and veterans' health centers.

Work hours vary, but nurses often need to work evening and weekend hours if employed in inpatient care centers.

Education and Training Requirements

- Must be currently licensed as an RN in the United States.
- Most often requires experience in both medical-surgical and mental health nursing.
- Must possess good interpersonal and communication skills.
- Should be compassionate and sympathetic toward this population.
- Background in psychology may be helpful.

Specialty Certification

Nurses can become nationally certified as a Certified Addictions Nurse through the Addictions Nursing Certification Board, part of the International Nurses Society on Addictions. To be eligible for certification, nurses should have a minimum of 2,000 hours of experience related to addictions care. Additionally, nurses should have 30 hours of continuing education in addictions nursing within the past 3 years.

Professional Organizations and Online Resources

International Nurses Society on Addictions: http://www.intnsa.org/certification

American Society of Addiction Medicine: http://www.asam.org/

Association for Addiction Professionals: http://www.naadac.org/

National Association of Addiction Treatment Providers: https://www.naatp.org/

#16

COMMUNITY HEALTH NURSE

Job Description

Community health nurses provide population-focused nursing care in a variety of settings. Community health nurses most often work in home healthcare agencies, but the term can be used broadly to define other nursing specialties, such as public, school, or occupational health nursing. Community health nurses provide holistic nursing care using the nursing process in settings where patients live, work, or congregate. They can provide direct or indirect care to individuals, families, and communities. Community health nursing care focuses on preserving, protecting, and promoting optimal health.

Typical Work Hours and Setting

Community health nurses can work in a variety of settings, depending on their focus of care. This can include home healthcare, schools, workplaces, health centers, health departments, congregations, and hospices. Work hours vary based on employment site, but community health nurses often need to work evening and weekend hours to accommodate the care of community-based patients.

Education and Training Requirements

- Must be currently licensed as an RN in the United States.
- Most often requires 1 to 2 years of acute care nursing experience.
- Should possess prior experience in a specific community health population (for instance, prior experience in pediatrics is required for school nursing).
- Must possess good interpersonal and communication skills.
- Should have good knowledge of community/ population of focus.
- Should be adaptable and flexible to work in various situations and settings.
- Must be able to promote culturally diverse nursing care.

Specialty Certification

Nurses can become nationally certified within several community health sub-specialties through the American Nurses Credentialing Center. While it no longer offers board certification in community health nursing, it has an advanced certification in public health. Nurses can check specific specialty associations to see whether they offer certification in their particular sub-specialty.

Professional Organizations and Online Resources

American Public Health Association: https://www.apha.org/

Association of Community Health Nursing Educators: http://www.achne.org/

Association of Public Health Nurses: http://www.phnurse.org/

American Nurses Credentialing Center: http://www.nursecredentialing.org/certification

#17

CORRECTIONAL NURSE

Job Description

Correctional nurses, or correctional facility nurses, provide care and support for inmates residing in facilities such as prisons, jails, penitentiaries, and juvenile homes. Correctional nurses must have good knowledge and skills in both acute and chronic medical conditions to provide comprehensive healthcare to a variety of inmates with various illnesses and injuries. In addition, nurses should have a good knowledge of mental health and substance abuse to care for the complex and diverse needs of the inmate population. Correctional nurses should be able to handle hostile situations in an environment that could potentially become violent or abusive.

Typical Work Hours and Setting

Correctional nurses work in inpatient correctional settings such as prisons and jails. Hours vary based on location and site, and some sites may require working evening, night, weekend, and holiday hours. Some correctional facilities that are part of a county, state, or the federal system often have very good benefits and an excellent compensation package.

Education and Training Requirements

- Must be currently licensed as an RN in the United States.
- Should have 1 to 2 years of acute care or mental health nursing experience.
- Must possess good interpersonal, communication, and teamwork skills.
- Should have experience working with diverse populations.
- Should be free of physical restrictions that can impede the ability to protect oneself in the event of an altercation with an inmate.

Specialty Certification

Nurses can become nationally certified as a Certified Correctional Health Professional Registered Nurse (CCHP-RN) through the National Commission on Correctional Health Care. To be eligible for the exam, nurses must have a minimum of working 2 years full time as a registered nurse, 2,000 hours working as a nurse in a correctional setting, and 54 hours of continuing education, with 18 hours in correctional healthcare within the last 3 years.

Professional Organizations and Online Resources

Correctional Nurse.net: http://correctionalnurse.net/

National Commission on Correctional Health Care: http://www.ncchc.org/

American Correctional Health Services Association: http://www.achsa.org/

American Correctional Association: http://www.aca.org/

Psychiatric RN

Tommy Williams, BSN, RN, CCHP

Q: What led you to your current career in nursing?

A: New nurses rarely get to choose what discipline they would like to practice in. It was simple need that led me to corrections—the jail needed a nurse and I needed a job. My goal was to get a year under my belt and then try to transition into psychiatric nursing. However, I found that I enjoyed working in corrections immensely. Because a large part of the incarcerated population also has some form of mental illness, most jails and prisons have a mental health team (including ours). Fortunately, the interest I expressed in transitioning from medical to psych was also shared by my employer.

Q: What are your typical job duties and responsibilities?

A: The primary duty of a correctional nurse is advocacy of inmates, and all responsibilities revolve around that. Specifically while working psych, I will do mental health (MH) intakes, follow-ups, respond to healthcare requests, and detox assessment. Interdisciplinary collaboration between the mental health team and correctional staff is evident in our daily meetings, where specific inmate needs and concerns are discussed. The initial MH intake helps me to determine what types of MH services might be required. I will collect collateral whenever possible. Any additional information gathered helps me to provide continuity of services and medications as best I can within institutional guidelines. Unfortunately, not all mentally ill inmates have an MH history in the community. Many suffer from anxiety or depression and up to the point of incarceration have self-medicated with illicit drugs and/or alcohol. Because of this, I try to explore non-pharmacological interventions that allow the individual to work through and resolve painful feelings instead of burying them with drugs. Supportive counseling is a big part of that process. If the inmate is displaying active symptoms of schizophrenia and appears to be a danger to themselves or others, I can place an MH hold on the individual and schedule an urgent assessment with a psychiatrist.

Q: Is there any special training or education required for your job?

A: Typical training (also common with most other nursing professions) includes BLS, infectious control/bloodborne pathogens, HIPPA, and OSHA. Specific to correctional nursing, PREA (Prison Rape Elimination Act) training must be completed every year. The CCHP (Certified Corrections Health Professional) certification is highly desired as it demonstrates mastery of national standards and knowledge expected of leaders working in this field. Also, mandatory training specific to each correctional facility is also required (typically some type of security training and protocols).

Q: What is the best part of your job?

A: While I primarily work as a psychiatric nurse, I often find myself using nursing skills from other specialties as well, including ED, med-surge, critical care, and any combination in between. Most get into nursing because they care for others and were looking for a profession that is representative of that desire. Correctional nursing is extremely rewarding and a satisfying experience as it requires care of a vulnerable population that have been removed from the rest of society.

Q: What is the least favorite part of your job?

A: My least favorite part of correctional nursing is trying to provide quality care in a place that was never designed for such. Nurses will work alongside corrections officers whose priorities of safety and security are different than patient-centered care and advocacy. This can occasionally cause tension due to the differences in approach. Additionally, because the correctional environment itself restricts freedom of movement, it can take considerable time to move just a short distance. The inability to navigate quickly within the institution is just accepted, and it isn't much of a problem—until a code is called.

Q: What advice would you give to those interested in pursuing a career in your nursing field?

A: Critical thinking, ability to prioritize, adaptability, and dependability are requisite traits. The commitment to the ethical provision of care to all individuals—regardless of the reason(s) for their incarceration—is crucial. It is necessary to have a "thick skin" and check your emotions at the gate. The population served typically will not recognize or appreciate the care you provide, and corrections staff sometimes perceive the nurse (especially new hires) as an outsider. Remind yourself that, at the end of the day, you get to go home to your family, decent meal, and soft bed.

Q: Anything important that you would like nurses to know about your nursing job?

A: Not at this time.

#18

DERMATOLOGY NURSE

Job Description

Dermatology nurses provide patients with the care of injuries and illnesses related to their skin. This includes management of various skin conditions, including wounds, psoriasis, eczema, acne, ulcers, and skin cancers. Additionally, some dermatology nurses may work in offices that offer cosmetic procedures and surgeries. The dermatology nurse will obtain a medical history and assessments; care for patients before, during, and after procedures; and provide education and discharge teaching regarding care of skin and wounds.

Typical Work Hours and Setting

Dermatology nurses usually work in outpatient dermatologist office settings and clinics. Some may also find employment in cosmetic surgery physician offices or centers. Typical hours are usually during normal business hours Monday through Friday unless required to participate in on-call hours.

Education and Training Requirements

- Must be currently licensed as an RN in the United States.
- Most often requires 1 to 2 years of prior nursing experience.
- Must possess good interpersonal and communication skills.
- Experience caring for patients with wounds is recommended.
- Should be able to care for patients with various stages and types of wounds.

Specialty Certification

Nurses can become nationally certified through the Dermatology Nurses' Association as a Dermatology Nurse Certified (DNC). To be eligible, nurses should have a minimum of 2 years experience as a registered nurse and a minimum of 2,000 hours working in dermatology.

Professional Organizations and Online Resources

Dermatology Nurses' Association:
http://www.dnanurse.org/

American Academy of Dermatology:
https://www.aad.org/

Wound, Ostomy and Continence Nurses Society:
http://www.wocn.org/

American Board of Dermatology:
https://www.abderm.org/

#19

DIABETES EDUCATOR NURSE

Job Description

The field of diabetes educator nursing is rapidly growing, and nurses are needed to help prevent new cases from occurring with the delivery of primary preventions and education. Diabetes educator nurses may engage in all aspects of the nursing process, including assessment of patients with diabetes and those who may be at risk, and implementation of diabetes management, including education about diet and medications and risks/complications associated with the disease. Nurses may also evaluate the plan of care and make changes to maximize optimal health and functioning for the patient with diabetes.

Typical Work Hours and Setting

Nurses who work as diabetes educators can work in both the inpatient and outpatient setting. Typical settings include medical offices and clinics that focus on the care of patients' diabetic/endocrine disorders. Home healthcare, public health, and long-term care are also settings that employ diabetes educator nurses. Work hours vary according to site but may most often be daytime hours Monday through Friday if within a medical office or clinic.

Education and Training Requirements

- Must be currently licensed as an RN in the United States.
- Most often requires prior knowledge and experience with the care of diabetic patients.
- Must possess good interpersonal and communication skills.
- Education experience is recommended.
- Should be knowledgeable with the management of both type I and II diabetes.

Specialty Certification

Nurses can become nationally certified as a Diabetes Educator (CNE) through the National Certification Board for Diabetes Educators. This certification is a practice-based one in which the candidate must demonstrate experience as a diabetes educator prior to obtaining certification. Certification is also available through the American Association of Diabetes Educators. However, that certification is limited to nurses who have a master's degree.

Professional Organizations and Online Resources

American Association of Diabetes Educators: https://www.diabeteseducator.org/

National Certification Board for Diabetes Educators: http://www.ncbde.org/

American Diabetes Association: http://www.diabetes.org/

DiabetesNet.com: http://www.diabetesnet.com/

20

DIALYSIS NURSE

Job Description

A dialysis nurse, also known as a *nephrology nurse,* works with patients who have inherited or acquired kidney diseases or abnormal kidney function that requires dialysis. Nurses provide care for patients who are undergoing dialysis treatments and provide care and education before, during, and after dialysis treatment. Dialysis nurses help provide education to patients on how to manage their disease and reduce complications, including teaching on diet/nutrition, medication management, and self-care strategies for chronic renal illness.

Typical Work Hours and Setting

Dialysis nurses can be employed in a variety of inpatient and outpatient settings, including acute/critical care settings, dialysis clinics, nephrology offices, home healthcare, and transplant units. Hours will vary according to the clinical site.

Education and Training Requirements

- Must be currently licensed as an RN in the United States.
- Most often requires 2 to 3 years of acute or critical care experience.

- Must possess good interpersonal and communication skills.
- Should possess good knowledge and skills pertaining to dialysis procedures and equipment.

Specialty Certification

Nurses can become nationally certified as a Certified Dialysis Nurse (CDN) through the Nephrology Nursing Certification Commission or the Board of Nephrology Examiners Nursing Technology. Both require experience and clinical hours working in the dialysis setting.

Professional Organizations and Online Resources

American Nephrology Nurses Association: https://www.annanurse.org/

Nephrology Nursing Certification Commission: https://www.nncc-exam.org/

National Kidney Foundation: https://www.kidney.org/

Board of Nephrology Examiners Nursing Technology: http://www.bonent.org/

#21

HOSPICE & PALLIATIVE CARE NURSE

Job Description

A hospice and palliative care nurse provides care to patients diagnosed with a life-threatening illness and their families. Using a palliative philosophy of care, nursing assessments and interventions are focused on providing comfort and improving quality of life. Hospice and palliative care nurses usually work as part of a team that includes other healthcare workers such as doctors, social workers, and chaplains. Patients are cared for holistically by focusing on physical, psychological, social, and spiritual aspects of care.

Typical Work Hours and Setting

Hospice and palliative care nurses can work in a home health agency and provide care for patients in their homes or in nursing homes. They can also work at freestanding inpatient hospices and comfort care homes. Work hours vary, but most case manager hospice nurses work Monday through Friday with some on-call responsibilities. Part-time or per diem hospice nurses can work on weekdays, weekends, and holidays.

Education and Training Requirements

- Requires an associate or baccalaureate degree in nursing.
- If hospice part of a home care agency, 1 to 2 years of basic home care experience is recommended.
- If position is part of a freestanding hospice, 2 to 3 years of acute care experience is preferred.
- Recommendation: Experience working in oncology (with cancer patients) may be beneficial in providing knowledge and skills in a type of illness that often precipitates hospice care.

Specialty Certification

Nurses can become nationally certified as a Certified Hospice and Palliative Nurse (CHPN) through the Hospice & Palliative Credentialing Center. Nurses must have a minimum of 500 hours of hospice and palliative care nursing practice to be eligible to sit for the exam.

Professional Organizations and Online Resources

Hospice & Palliative Nurses Association:
http://hpna.advancingexpertcare.org/

Hospice & Palliative Credentialing Center:
http://hpcc.advancingexpertcare.org/

American Academy of Hospice and Palliative Medicine:
http://aahpm.org/

National Hospice and Palliative Care Organization:
http://www.nhpco.org/

career highlight

Hospice & Palliative Care Nurse

Susan Lowey, RN, CHPN

Q: What led you to your current career in nursing?

A: Before I was a hospice nurse, I worked in the hospital, nursing home, and in home healthcare. I have always been interested in caring for patients who were living with serious illnesses and felt drawn to be there for them. I enjoy talking with patients and their families and listening to their concerns. At the time I started my career in hospice, I was a registered nurse with a bachelor's degree but since then have gone on to receive advanced graduate degrees. I worked as a nursing assistant for 7 years and then as a nurse for 5 years before I started working in hospice care. I was working in home healthcare and had many patients with serious illnesses who ended up dying. I enjoyed the care that I gave them towards the end of their lives and felt that I really made a difference for them. That is what led me to pursue a job in hospice care.

Q: What are your typical job duties and responsibilities?

A: As a hospice nurse in home healthcare, I make home visits to provide care to patients and their families. I evaluate patients for hospice eligibility, admit patients to home hospice care, and make visits to the home to assess patients for response to the hospice interdisciplinary plan of care. This includes assessment of symptoms and the patient's response to management, psychosocial and spiritual assessment, evaluation of the patient's goals of care, emotional support for the patient and family, education about medications and the comfort-oriented plan of care, and education about the dying process and grief. I also make home visits after a hospice patient has died and offer support to the family, contact the appropriate persons, and pronounce the patient's death. I participate in interdisciplinary team meetings and precept new nurses and nursing students.

Q: Is there any special training or education required for your job?

A: I have several years of acute care experience prior to working in home healthcare. I worked in home care for a few years before starting work in hospice. The acute care and home care experience were both beneficial for preparing me for working in home hospice care. I was pursuing graduate education during much of the time I was working in hospice care, so that focused education in end-of-life and palliative care helped me to develop my skills in hospice care. I also joined the Hospice & Palliative Nurses Association and became specialty certified through the Hospice & Palliative Credentialing Center, both of which helped me to further develop a comprehensive skill set for my role as a hospice and palliative care nurse.

Q: What is the best part of your job?

A: Knowing that I make a difference in the lives of patients who are dying is the best part of my job. I enjoy being able to lessen their pain or other adverse symptoms associated with the dying process. I also enjoy being able to provide emotional and spiritual support for patients and their families throughout their personal journeys. It is truly an honor to be able to be with patients throughout their final journey in life.

Q: What is the least favorite part of your job?

A: The least favorite part of my job is knowing that most of my patients will die and that my time with them will be limited. The other least favorite part is having to inform family members that their loved one is very close to death so they can prepare in whatever ways they need to (i.e., contact clergy or other family members who want to be present).

Q: What advice would you give to those interested in pursuing a career in your nursing field?

A: In order to be a good hospice nurse, you must have excellent communication skills, you must be comfortable talking with people about sensitive topics, comfortable talking to people about spiritual concerns and needs, and be able to cope with multiple losses of patients as part of your daily job. I would also suggest that anyone interested in hospice nursing may want to work in oncology with cancer patients initially to see if they like the work involved with that patient population. Since many hospice patients have a cancer diagnosis, prior experience with cancer nursing would be helpful.

Q: Anything important that you would like nurses to know about your nursing job?

A: I don't want nurses to think that working with patients who are dying is depressing and difficult to do. It is not easy at times to deal with multiple losses of patients and to witness patients during difficult times and those in pain or suffering. But the work that hospice nurses do to bring comfort and help patients find peace occurs more so than the negative aspects. I wouldn't have been able to stay as long in hospice as I have if it was not a personally and professionally rewarding nursing career. I honestly cannot think of any other patient population who I would enjoy working with as much as the patients I care for. I am glad to be there for patients and families often, during their darkest hour.

22

NURSE CASE MANAGER

Job Description

The primary role of a nurse case manager is to organize, co-ordinate, and manage the care needs of his or her patient population and setting. The main goal of the nurse case manager role is to promote cost-effective continuity of care along the illness trajectory for patients. Case manager nurses may work with a variety of patients along the age or illness continuum in a variety of care settings. The focus is on the individual patient. Nurse case managers should have excellent organizational and analytic skills to evaluate a quality plan of care for patients.

Typical Work Hours and Setting

Nurse case managers can work in a variety of settings with diverse patient populations. They can work in both inpatient and outpatient settings in home health agencies, physician offices, medical clinics, hospices, rehabilitation facilities, occupational health, and long-term care and managed-care organizations.

Education and Training Requirements

- Must be currently licensed as an RN in the United States.
- Most often requires previous nursing experience.
- Must possess excellent interpersonal, communication, and negotiation skills.
- Should possess knowledge about the resources available in the community.
- Must be able to work well in an interdisciplinary setting.

Specialty Certification

Nurse case managers can become board certified through the Commission for Case Manager Certification as a Certified Case Manager (CCM). To be eligible, nurses should have their RN license and have a baccalaureate degree. They must also have 12 to 24 months of experience in case management.

Professional Organizations and Online Resources

Commission for Case Manager Certification: https://ccmcertification.org/

American Case Management Association: http://www.acmaweb.org/

Case Management Society of America: http://www.cmsa.org/

National Registered Nurse Case Manager Training Center: https://nationalrncasemanagertraining.com/

#23

OCCUPATIONAL HEALTH NURSE

Job Description

Occupational, or environmental, health nurses monitor and implement health and safety services to workers in various employment settings. The goal is to promote worker population health and reduce or prevent illness or injury, specifically work-related or environmental hazards. Depending on the role, occupational health nurses' responsibilities may include coordination of workers' compensation, short- and long-term disability, and the Family Medical Leave Act (FMLA). Some may be involved in managing compliance issues related to state and federal regulations, such as the Occupational Safety and Health Administration (OSHA), and tracking or monitoring workplace incidents and injuries. Disaster and emergency planning and management is another part of the occupational health nurse role.

Typical Work Hours and Setting

Occupational health nurses can work in any type of employment setting, including manufacturing and production, healthcare facilities and medical centers, and any other employment sector. Hours will vary according to specific site.

Education and Training Requirements

- Must be currently licensed as an RN in the United States.
- Baccalaureate degree is most preferred.
- Should have knowledge of OSHA regulations.
- Must have strong communication and organizational skills.
- Should be able to provide health and safety educational training to the worker population.

Specialty Certification

Nurses can become nationally certified in occupational health through the American Board for Occupational Health Nurses and receive the Certified Occupational Health Nurse (COHN) credential. To be eligible, nurses must have worked 3,000 hours within the last 5 years in an occupational health setting. Nurses may also pursue certification as a Certified Occupational Health Nurse Specialist (COHN-S), which requires a baccalaureate degree in addition to practice hours.

Professional Organizations and Online Resources

American Association of Occupational Health Nurses: http://aaohn.org/

American Board for Occupational Health Nurses, Inc: https://www.abohn.org/

Association of Occupational Health Professionals in Healthcare: https://www.aohp.org/

#24

ONCOLOGY NURSE

Job Description

Oncology nurses provide nursing care across the continuum for patients with cancer. Nurses provide health education and care to reduce risks for developing cancer, assist in the diagnostic modalities used to diagnose cancer, and implement interventions to treat cancer. Oncology nurses provide counseling and emotional support for patients and their families who are undergoing a cancer diagnosis and treatment. The oncology nurse can specialize in a specific patient population, such as pediatric, or in a specific type of cancer, such as solid tumor. Nurses can also specialize in a specific type of treatment for cancer, such as in chemotherapy, radiation, or surgery.

Typical Work Hours and Setting

Oncology nurses can work in a variety of inpatient and outpatient settings. This includes cancer treatment centers, oncologist offices, radiation clinics, outpatient chemotherapy oncology centers, home healthcare, pain management clinics, and hospice/palliative care.

Education and Training Requirements

- Must be currently licensed as an RN in the United States.
- Must possess good understanding of cancer care.
- Must possess good interpersonal and communication skills.
- Must possess sensitivity and be able to provide support for patients and families.
- Should be willing to keep abreast of new interventions and therapies used to detect and treat cancer.

Specialty Certification

Nurses can become nationally certified as an Oncology Certified Nurse (OCN) through the Oncology Nursing Certification Corporation. Nurses must have a minimum of 1 year of nursing experience with at least 1,000 practice hours in oncology nursing and 10 continuing education hours in oncology. The Oncology Nursing Certification Corporation offers several other sub-specialty oncology nurse certifications.

Professional Organizations and Online Resources

Oncology Nursing Society: https://www.ons.org/

Oncology Nursing Certification Corporation: http://www.oncc.org/

International Society of Nurses in Cancer Care: http://www.isncc.org/

Association of Pediatric Hematology/Oncology Nurses: http://www.aphon.org/

#25

PUBLIC HEALTH NURSE

Job Description

Public health nurses help prevent illnesses and injury in the population they serve through primary, secondary, and tertiary preventions. Public health nurses can provide care for individuals, families, groups, and communities through preventative programs, education, screenings, implementation of programs and interventions, community assessments and program planning, research, and policy initiatives. Emergency and disaster preparedness may also be part of the role of some nurses working in public health.

Typical Work Hours and Setting

Public health nurses can work in county, state, or federal health departments and agencies and can specialize in sub-specialties such as immunization, tuberculosis, sexually transmitted disease, infectious diseases, smoking cessation, teen pregnancy, poverty and homelessness, migrant care, etc. Work hours will vary according to job description and type. Some travel to homes or other sites to provide care may be required.

Education and Training Requirements

- Must be currently licensed as an RN in the United States.
- Most often requires a baccalaureate degree in nursing.
- Must possess good interpersonal, communication, and problem solving skills.
- Should have training in the delivery of cultural competent and sensitive care.
- Should possess good knowledge of the population they are serving.

Specialty Certification

The American Nurses Credentialing Center has retired its public health nursing certification exam. Nurses who seek certification in public health may do so through the National Board of Public Health Examiners for a Certified Public Health (CPH) credential. To be eligible, nurses must possess a bachelor's degree and a minimum of 5 years experience working in public health.

Professional Organizations and Online Resources

Association of Public Health Nurses: http://www.phnurse.org/

American Public Health Association: https://www.apha.org/

National Board of Public Health Examiners: https://www.nbphe.org/

Quad Council Coalition: http://www.quadcouncilphn.org/

Tuberculosis Case Manager

Renee Jenkins, BSN, RN

Q: What led you to your current career in nursing?

A: I wanted a change in the type of nursing I was previously doing yet wanted to continue to be an advocate and educator for patients. Here in this clinic, I get to do all of that and more. I learn and teach about diversity, precept nursing students, educate the public about tuberculosis, and collaborate and consult with physicians and residents.

Q: What are your typical job duties and responsibilities?

A: Opening new cases of patients with tuberculosis, especially when the patient is still in the hospital setting. Collect specimens such as blood draws and sputum for diagnostic testing and continued monitoring; review laboratory results, interview patients, obtain health history, and complete patient assessments.

Q: Is there any special training or education required for your job?

A: No; however, good interpersonal skills are an asset. A public speaking class would also be beneficial.

Q: What is the best part of your job?

A: Knowing that I am helping to make my community safe. I feel successful when patients complete their course of treatment.

Q: What is the least favorite part of your job?

A: The least favorite part of my job is having to place PPDs (skin testing for TB) on small infants and children.

Q: What advice would you give to those interested in pursuing a career in your nursing field?

A: Have a love of people! Have a great sense of humor. Know the difference between sympathy and empathy. Enjoy working with different cultures and nationalities.

Q: Anything important that you would like nurses to know about your nursing job?

A: A public health/community health nurse must know how to work independent of a physician yet remain within the scope of RN practice. A class or independent reading on role structure, group dynamics, and cultural diversity would help to understand and appreciate other cultures. It is also important to realize that what is acceptable or not acceptable in our own community/culture may or may not be the norm in other communities/cultures. Thus, a public health nurse cannot be judgmental but can offer assistance.

#26

RADIOLOGY NURSE

Job Description

A radiology nurse provides care to patients who are under-going diagnostic or therapeutic radiology procedures. This can includes patients with cancer who receive radiology treatments to eradicate cancer cells or patients who are undergoing an MRI to diagnose a condition. Radiology nurses use medical technology equipment in their daily work and care of patients. They perform assessments and obtain health history, provide medications and care for pa-tients during the procedure, and monitor patients post pro-cedure for complications. Radiology nurses must have a good knowledge of radiation treatment and safety.

Typical Work Hours and Setting

Radiology nurses can work in both inpatient and outpatient settings. This can include radiology departments and cen-ters, endoscopy clinics, nuclear medicine, and surgical and cancer treatment centers. Hours will be mainly business hours Monday through Friday unless on-call or off shifts are required.

Education and Training Requirements

- Must be currently licensed as an RN in the United States.
- Should have 2 to 3 years of experience in medical sur-gical nursing or acute care.
- Must possess good interpersonal and communication skills.
- Should have good working knowledge of technology and information systems.
- Should be able to work in a fast-paced environment alongside an interdisciplinary team.

Specialty Certification

Nurses can become nationally certified as a Certified Radiology Nurse (CRN) through the Radiologic Nursing Certification Board. To be eligible, nurses must have a minimum of 2,000 hours in radiology nursing within the past 3 years and have obtained a minimum of 30 continuing education hours in radiology nursing over the past 24 months.

Professional Organizations and Online Resources

Association for Radiologic & Imaging Nursing:
http://arinursing.org/

Radiologic Nursing Certification Board:
https://www.certifiedradiologynurse.org

Society of Interventional Radiology:
http://www.sirweb.org/

American Society for Therapeutic Radiation Oncology:
https://www.astro.org/home/

#27

REHABILITATION NURSE

Job Description

Rehabilitation nurses assist patients with acute or chronic illnesses and disabilities to restore optimal functioning and improve quality of life. Rehabilitation nurses help to plan and develop a plan of care that promotes patients in self-care and optimal recovery of their condition. They can assist patients with long-term care planning and securing resources for care if required. Nurses help patients to regain as much independence as possible while providing safe holistic care during their recovery. Patients can be any age along the life span; however, working with the adult and older adult population is typical.

Typical Work Hours and Setting

Rehabilitation nurses can work in both inpatient and outpatient care settings. They can work in rehabilitation facilities and clinics, long-term care and assisted living centers, home healthcare, hospices, and pain management clinics. They can work in acute or chronic care facilities. Work hours vary according to the site but may include evening, night, or weekend hours in inpatient facilities.

Education and Training Requirements

- Must be currently licensed as an RN in the United States.
- Most often requires 1 to 2 years of acute care or medical surgical experience.
- Must possess good interpersonal, communication, and organizational skills.
- Should be able to provide emotional support for patients and families.
- Should have good knowledge of resources in the area for patient care planning.

Specialty Certification

Nurses can become nationally certified as a Certified Rehabilitation Registered nurse (CRRN) through the Association of Rehabilitation Nurses. To be eligible, nurses must have 2 years of practice as a registered nurse in rehabilitation nursing within the past 5 years or have 1 year of rehabilitation nursing and 1 year of advanced nursing study beyond the baccalaureate degree level.

Professional Organizations and Online Resources

Association of Rehabilitation Nurses: http://www.rehabnurse.org/

International Association of Rehabilitation Professionals: http://www.rehabpro.org/

National Rehabilitation Association: https://www.nationalrehab.org/

United Spinal Association: http://www.spinalcord.org/

#28

UROLOGY NURSE

Job Description

Urology nurses care for patients who have illnesses or injuries related to the urinary system. Some of these conditions could include cancer, urinary tract infections, and issues with continence. Nurses must be prepared to care for patients who are dealing with discomfort and embarrassment. Typical job responsibilities may include assessment and patient history, collection of urine specimens, patient teaching regarding urology health, and implantation of treatments for urinary disorders.

Typical Work Hours and Setting

Urology nurses can work in both inpatient and outpatient settings. This can include urology offices and clinics, physician and geriatrician offices, and in long-term care or assisted living centers. Work hours may vary according to clinical site.

Education and Training Requirements

- Must be currently licensed as an RN in the United States.
- Most often requires 1 to 2 years of medical surgical experience.

- Should possess good knowledge of the urinary and reproductive systems.
- Should have good communication and interpersonal skills.
- Should possess sensitivity related to urinary issues.

Specialty Certification

Nurses can become nationally certified as a Certified Urologic Registered Nurse (CURN) through the Certification Board for Urologic Nurses and Associates. To be eligible, nurses should have a minimum of 2 years' experience working as a registered nurse with a minimum of 800 clinical hours working in urology. Depending on job role, nurses may choose to become certified as a Wound, Ostomy, and Continence Nurse (WOCN) through the Wound, Ostomy and Continence Nurses Society.

Professional Organizations and Online Resources

Society of Urologic Nurses and Associates: https://www.suna.org/

Certification Board for Urologic Nurses and Associates: https://www.cbuna.org/

American Urological Association: https://www.auanet.org/

Urology Care Foundation: http://www.urologyhealth.org/

Wound, Ostomy and Continence Nurses Society: http://www.wocn.org/

PART 4

OLDER ADULTS

#29

ADULT DAY PROGRAM NURSE

Job Description

Adult day program nurses provide care for residents of adult day programs. Patients may most often be older adults but may also include younger adults with physical or mental disabilities that require day program care. Responsibilities can include patient assessments, triage of patient concerns or issues, administration of medication and treatments, assistance with activities of daily living, and engagement with residents in social therapies and programs. Nurses frequently collaborate and engage with various other team members in the care of residents.

Typical Work Hours and Setting

Adult day program nurses usually work in outpatient care programs that may or may not be associated with medical centers, home healthcare agencies, or long-term care facilities. Work hours will typically be during business hours Monday through Friday unless the program includes weekend hours.

Education and Training Requirements

- Must be currently licensed as an RN in the United States.
- Most often requires 1 to 2 years of experience working with older or disabled adults.
- Must possess good interpersonal and communication skills.
- Should be sensitive to the needs and concerns of chronically ill patients.

Specialty Certification

Although there is no specific certification for adult day program nursing, nurses may become board certified in gerontological nursing through the American Nurses Credentialing Center.

Professional Organizations and Online Resources

American Nurses Credentialing Center:
http://www.nursecredentialing.org/

Gerontological Society of America:
https://www.geron.org/

National Gerontological Nursing Association:
http://www.ngna.org/

#30

ASSISTED LIVING NURSE

Job Description

Assisted living nurses may have several different roles and responsibilities. Some of these may include administrative, case management, and care coordination duties, such as admission of new residents and oversight of existing residents in the facility. Other roles may be more clinically oriented, including hands-on care, medication management, triage and assessment of residents, and on-call duties as needed. Assisted living nurses work with residents and their families in developing a feasible plan of care for residents that meet their goals of care.

Typical Work Hours and Setting

Assisted living nurses may only work business hours Monday through Friday if primarily in an administrative position. Nurses working in a clinical role may work evening, weekend, and on-call hours to meet the needs of residents.

Education and Training Requirements

- Must be currently licensed as an RN in the United States.
- Most often requires 1 to 2 years of experience working with older or disabled adults.
- Must possess good interpersonal and communication skills.
- Should be sensitive to the needs and concerns of chronically ill patients.

Specialty Certification

Nurses can become specialty certified as a Certified Assisted Living Nurse through the American Assisted Living Nurses Association. Nurses with current experience working in assisted living are eligible to apply.

Professional Organizations and Online Resources

American Assisted Living Nurses Association: https://www.alnursing.org/

National Center for Assisted Living: https://www.ahcancal.org/ncal/pages/index.aspx

National Gerontological Nursing Association: http://www.ngna.org/

Gerontological Society of America: https://www.geron.org/

#31

CARDIOPULMONARY REHABILITATION NURSE

Job Description

Cardiopulmonary rehabilitation nurses are vital in improving the outcomes of patients with acute and chronic conditions of the heart and lungs. Nurses help assess and implement cardiopulmonary rehab with patients who are in various stages of their illness. Cardiopulmonary rehab nurses must possess an excellent understanding of cardiac health, and previous experience in cardiology is required. Nurses assess and monitor patients during rehabilitation treatments and provide education about lifestyle changes. They often must deal with patients who do not embrace or follow the lifestyle changes that are being encouraged; however, providing a supportive health environment for patients throughout the process is crucial.

Typical Work Hours and Setting

Cardiopulmonary rehab nurses can work in both inpatient and outpatient settings. Most often, they are employed in ambulatory cardiac centers or heart failure, pulmonary, or exercise physiology clinics. They can also work in physician or cardiology practices. Some may even find employment in fitness gyms. Work hours vary according to site but often follow normal business hours Monday through Friday.

Education and Training Requirements

- Must be currently licensed as an RN in the United States.
- Should have 3 to 4 years of experience as an RN in acute cardiac or critical care.
- Must possess good assessment and critical thinking skills.
- Should have a good understanding of cardiac health and exercise physiology.
- Should have excellent communication skills and a desire to teach health promotion.

Specialty Certification

Nurses can become nationally certified as a Certified Cardiac Rehabilitation Professional and earn the CCRP credential through the American Association of Cardiovascular and Pulmonary Rehabilitation. To be eligible, nurses must have a minimum of 1,200 clinical hours in cardiac rehab/secondary prevention. A baccalaureate degree in nursing is preferred.

Professional Organizations and Online Resources

American Association of Cardiovascular and Pulmonary Rehabilitation: https://www.aacvpr.org/

American Board of Cardiovascular Medicine: http://www.abcmcertification.com/

Preventive Cardiovascular Nurses Association: http://pcna.net/

American Heart Association: http://www.heart.org/HEARTORG/

career highlight

Cardiology Practice Nurse

Kathleen R. Ross, BSN, RN

Q: What led you to your current career in nursing?

A: My current job in cardiac rehab came out of the critical care unit (CCU) that I worked in. The CCU staff was allowed to be part of the team that started cardiac rehab. Our cardiac rehab was the first one developed in the local area. I did work on that committee. I worked per diem after my rotation. I was also looking to get off of weekends when I transferred to rehab. I loved my CCU job; however, I needed more regular hours so our children would have a parent at their sporting events.

Q: What are your typical job duties and responsibilities?

A: We are responsible to oversee the safe exercise of all the cardiac rehab and pulmonary rehab patients. An RN must be in the department for any patient to exercise. Any medical issues are run through the RN to triage, and if it is an actual problem, we handle it. We either call the patient's doctor, our physician on-call, or 911 or hospital, depending on the urgency of the problem. We call patients to schedule their intake interview, and set up patient exercise schedules and/or follow-up appointments that are needed to keep patients moving forward in rehab. We do primary care so who initially interviews the patient is responsible for that patient through discharge. If an exercise physiologist's patient has an issue, an RN usually has to contact the physician, as they cannot take phone orders for medication changes at times the nurse may need to take over the care of the patient if needed. Patient education is a big part of what we offer. We have group classes and we also do a lot of one-on-one education. Lots of blood pressure monitoring.

Q: Is there any special training or education required for your job?

A: Registered nurses in cardiopulmonary rehab should have the following:

- ICU/critical care background, 2 to 3 years preferred.
- Telemetry experience a minimum; pass a telemetry class.
- Must be ACLS & BLS certified within a year of starting in rehab if you don't have it when you start.

Q: What is the best part of your job?

A: The patients; seeing a patient who comes in with low functioning leave rehab being able to do some things they never thought they could ever do again; helping patients and families understand what happened to them; after teaching an educational class, having a patient come up and tell you what a great class you just taught. Many of the patients become family.

Q: What is the least favorite part of your job?

A: The least favorite part of my job is also the patients. At times they are very demanding and not very understanding that medicine is not an exact science and that there are not always answers for why something went this way or not. Getting a patient or family to understand that they caused some of their problems and not always that someone did something wrong. And the computer—it hates me!

Q: What advice would you give to those interested in pursuing a career in your nursing field?

A: Get experience in critical care and/or cardiology. This will help you when you are triaging a patient complaint. If able to take an exercise science class, that would help you better understand the physiology of exercise. I call it the twinkle in their eye. You have to be able to tell when their complaints are important and may need a physician follow-up or to be sent to the emergency department (ED). Patients and physicians don't like it when you send everyone to the ED that could be handled at home or in their office. I call it identifying that twinkle in their eye, something seriously wrong but not a lot of data to tell you what.

Q: Anything important that you would like nurses to know about your nursing job?

A: If you don't like to work independently and need supervision or guidance, this may not be for you. The RN is who the rest of the staff, and at times the other RNs, look to in order to keep patients safe. If you don't like to teach you may want to go into a different job. Lastly, you need to accept that not all patients will listen to your advice or suggestions and will do what they want, even if it isn't in their best interest. You can't change the world, only educate them and hope they make the right changes.

32

GERIATRIC NURSE

Job Description

Geriatric nurses provide comprehensive and holistic nursing care to the older adult population. They must focus on restoring or maintaining the physiological and psychological health and functioning of elderly patients. The goal is to assist patients to achieve or maintain an optimal level of functioning that is aligned with their goals of care to promote their quality of life. Patients often have complex care needs that impact more than just physical functioning, and nurses should be skilled in the assessment and management of psychological, emotional, social, cultural, and spiritual health of a growing older adult population. Geriatric nurses should be knowledgeable in cognitive disorders, such as Alzheimer's disease, medication management, poly-pharmacy, self-care strategies, management of chronic illness, environmental safety concerns, and sleep and sexual concerns.

Typical Work Hours and Setting

Geriatric nurses can work in both inpatient and outpatient care settings. They can work in long-term care facilities, such as nursing homes and assisted living centers, adult day care programs, senior centers, community health centers and clinics, home healthcare agencies, transitional care centers, and physician and geriatrician offices.

Education and Training Requirements

- Must be currently licensed as an RN in the United States.
- Most often requires 1 to 2 years of experience working with older adults.
- Must possess good interpersonal and communication skills.
- Should have sensitivity and patience with the needs and concerns of elderly patients.
- Must be able and willing to advocate for older adults with physical and cognitive impairments.

Specialty Certification

Nurses can become board certified in gerontological nursing earning an RN-BC credential through the American Nurses Credentialing Center. To be eligible, nurses must have a minimum of 2 years experience as a registered nurse, 2,000 hours of clinical practice, and 30 hours of continuing education in gerontological nursing.

Professional Organizations and Online Resources

National Gerontological Nursing Association: http://www.ngna.org/

American Nurses Credentialing Center: http://www.nursecredentialing.org/certification

American Geriatrics Society: http://www.americangeriatrics.org/

Gerontological Society of America: https://www.geron.org/

#33

GERO-PSYCHIATRIC NURSE

Job Description

Gero-psychiatric nurses care for older adults with mental health disorders. This can include depression, anxiety, bipolar disorder, schizophrenia, delirium, dementia, and addictions. This sub-specialty is a mix between geriatric and mental health nursing. Gero-psychiatric nurses must possess excellent communication skills and sensitivity to this special-needs population. Nurses use the nursing process in the assessment, implementation, and evaluation of patients receiving treatment for mental health disorders. The gero-psychiatric nurse provides education and support to patients and families. They may participate in or lead individual or group counseling sessions, provide information regarding community resources, and plan for long-term care needs.

Typical Work Hours and Setting

Although many gero-psychiatric nurse positions are located in the inpatient setting, nurses can work in community and ambulatory-based senior care centers, home healthcare, elderly advocacy and abuse coalitions, managed care, insurance companies, and gero-psychiatry offices. Some mental health facilities or emergency departments may offer positions for gero-psychiatric nurses.

Education and Training Requirements

- Must be currently licensed as an RN in the United States.
- Should have prior experience working with the geriatric and/or psychiatric population.
- Must possess excellent interpersonal, listening, and communication skills.
- Must be able to foster a therapeutic and trustworthy relationship with patients.
- Should have sensitivity and patience with the needs and concerns of elderly patients.
- Must be able to advocate for the needs of this patient population.

Specialty Certification

Although there is currently no board certification awarded for gero-psychiatric nursing, nurses can choose to become certified in gerontological nursing or psychiatric-mental health nursing or both, through the American Nurses Credentialing Center.

Professional Organizations and Online Resources

American Nurses Credentialing Center: http://www.nursecredentialing.org/

National Gerontological Nursing Association: http://www.ngna.org/

American Psychiatric Nurses Association: http://www.apna.org/

American Association for Geriatric Psychiatry: http://www.aagponline.org/

#34

LONG-TERM CARE NURSE

Job Description

Long-term care nurses provide comprehensive and holistic nursing care to the older adult population residing in long-term care facilities. This can include nursing homes, assisted living facilities, and hospices. Nurses focus on the care of elderly residents' physiological and psychological health and functioning. Typical duties may include assessments of residents, triaging resident complaints, administration of medications and treatments, continual evaluation of resident plan of care, and supervision of unlicensed healthcare personnel.

Typical Work Hours and Setting

Long-term care nurses typically work in a nursing home or an assisted living facility. Their work hours may vary and could include evening, nights, and weekend hours. Many long-term care facilities employ registered nurses for charge, supervisor, or nurse manager positions. Hours will vary according to the specific role and responsibility of the nurse. Other long-term care nursing settings may include home health and/or hospice care.

Education and Training Requirements

- Must be currently licensed as an RN in the United States.
- Most often requires 1 to 2 years of experience working with older adults.
- Must possess good interpersonal and communication skills.
- Should have sensitivity and patience with the needs and concerns of elderly patients.
- Must be able and willing to advocate for older adults with physical and cognitive impairments.

Specialty Certification

There is currently no specific board certification for nurses in long-term care. However, nurses can become board certified in gerontological nursing earning an RN-BC credential through the American Nurses Credentialing Center. To be eligible, nurses must have a minimum of 2 years of experience as a registered nurse, 2,000 hours of clinical practice, and 30 hours of continuing education in gerontological nursing.

Professional Organizations and Online Resources

National Long Term Care Network: http://nltcn.com/

National Association for the Support of Long Term Care: https://www.nasl.org/

National Gerontological Nursing Association: http://www.ngna.org/

Leading Age (formerly American Association of Homes and Services for the Aging): http://www.leadingage.org/

#35

LONG-TERM CARE NURSE SUPERVISOR

Job Description

Long-term care nurse supervisors provide oversight and supervision of licensed and unlicensed healthcare staff working in long-term care facilities. This can include nursing homes, assisted living facilities, and hospices. Nurses focus on ensuring the delivery of quality physiological and psychological care for elderly residents living in long-term care. Long-term care nurse supervisors may have administrative duties ensuring adequate staffing is met, which may include coordination of supplemental agency staffing. They may also be responsible for completing and/or oversight of collection of the long-term care minimal data set (MDS) data required from all residents who are Medicare beneficiaries who reside in a nursing home.

Typical Work Hours and Setting

Long-term care nurses typically work in a nursing home or assisted living facility. Their work hours may vary and could include evening, nights, and weekend hours. Many long-term care facilities employ registered nurses for charge, supervisor, or nurse manager positions. Hours will vary according to the specific role and responsibility of the nurse. Other long-term care nursing settings may include home health and/or hospice care.

Education and Training Requirements

- Must be currently licensed as an RN in the United States.
- Most often requires 1 to 2 years of experience working with older adults.
- Must possess good interpersonal and communication skills.
- Should have sensitivity and patience with the needs and concerns of elderly patients.
- Must be able and willing to advocate for older adults with physical and cognitive impairments.

Specialty Certification

There is currently no specific board certification for nurses in long-term care. However, nurses can become board certified in gerontological nursing earning an RN-BC credential through the American Nurses Credentialing Center. To be eligible, nurses must have a minimum of 2 years experience as a registered nurse, 2,000 hours of clinical practice, and 30 hours of continuing education in gerontological nursing.

Professional Organizations and Online Resources

National Long Term Care Network: http://nltcn.com/

National Association for the Support of Long Term Care: https://www.nasl.org/

National Gerontological Nursing Association: http://www.ngna.org/

Leading Age (formerly American Association of Homes and Services for the Aging): http://www.leadingage.org/

#36

TELEMEDICINE NURSE

Job Description

Telemedicine, or telehealth nursing, is an emerging field. Telemedicine nurses use various technology to provide nursing care to patients in various settings. This can include the use of audio, video, or remote data of patients delivered electronically. Many home health agencies have telemedicine departments that utilize telemedicine with the routine monitoring of some of their patients. This can include patients living with chronic conditions and also patients living in distant rural settings. Telemedicine nurses should be knowledgeable about the use of technology to deliver care to patients.

Typical Work Hours and Setting

Telemedicine nurses can work in a variety of outpatient settings, including home healthcare, physician offices, medical clinics, and telemedicine centers. Their work hours vary according to site. Most nurses work out of an office with the remote monitoring of patients in distant settings.

Education and Training Requirements

- Must be currently licensed as an RN in the United States.
- Most often requires 2 to 3 years of previous nursing experience.
- Must possess good interpersonal, listening, and communication skills.
- Must be able to manage informational systems and electronic medical technology.
- Should have strong computer skills.

Specialty Certification

Although there is no current specific nursing certification for telemedicine, nurses can become certified in ambulatory care and receive the RN-BC designation through the American Nurses Credentialing Center. To be eligible, nurses must have been in practice as a registered nurse for a minimum of 2 years full time, have worked 2,000 hours in ambulatory care and/or telehealth nursing, and have completed 30 hours of continuing education in ambulatory care or telehealth.

Professional Organizations and Online Resources

American Telemedicine Association:
http://www.americantelemed.org/

Telemedicine Nursing Fact Sheet:
http://www.americantelemed.org/docs/default-document-library/fact_sheet_final.pdf?sfvrsn=2

International Society for Telemedicine and eHealth:
https://www.isfteh.org/

American Academy of Ambulatory Care Nursing:
https://www.aaacn.org/telehealth

37

WOUND, OSTOMY, & CONTINENCE NURSE

Job Description

Wound, ostomy, & continence nurses care for patients who have the presence of wounds, colostomies, or urinary issues with incontinence. Nurses must be prepared to care for patients who are dealing with discomfort and embarrassment. Typical job responsibilities may include assessment and patient history, collection of specimens, and patient teaching regarding skin, wound care, ostomy, and genitourinary care. These nurses are specialists in the care and management of the latest interventions used to manage these medical conditions. They are often sought out as a resource in healthcare organizations by staff caring for patients with wound, ostomy, or continence needs.

Typical Work Hours and Setting

Wound, ostomy, & continence nurses can work in many different inpatient and outpatient settings, including physician offices and clinics, long-term care or assisted living centers, wound treatment clinics, urologist offices, and home healthcare. Work hours may vary according to clinical site.

Education and Training Requirements

- Must be currently licensed as an RN in the United States.
- Most often requires 1 to 2 years of medical surgical experience.
- Should possess good knowledge of the gastrointestinal, genitourinary, and/or integumentary systems.
- Should have good communication and interpersonal skills.
- Should possess sensitivity related to issues associated with the presence of wounds, ostomies, and incontinence.

Specialty Certification

Nurses can become nationally certified as a Wound, Ostomy, and Continence Nurse (WOCN) through the Wound, Ostomy and Continence Nurses Society. There are two pathways to become eligible to obtain this certification. One is the traditional pathway in which nurses must graduate from an accredited WOC nursing program. The other pathway involves obtaining a minimum of 1,500 direct clinical patient care hours in WOC nursing in addition to 50 continuing education credits in wound, ostomy, and continence nursing.

Professional Organizations and Online Resources

Wound, Ostomy and Continence Nurses Society: http://www.wocn.org/

Wound, Ostomy and Continence Nursing Certification Board: https://www.wocncb.org/

Society of Urologic Nurses and Associates: https://www.suna.org/

American Urological Association: https://www.auanet.org/

International Continence Society: http://www.ics.org/

PART **5**

OTHER NON-HOSPITAL NURSING CAREERS

#38

ARMED FORCES MILITARY NURSE

Job Description

Military nurses care for patients and their families who are members of the armed forces. They can be stationed to work at military bases in the United States or may be deployed to work abroad, particularly in times of active war. Typical duties include providing routine and entry health screenings, ongoing monitoring of health conditions, triage and acute care of injuries and illnesses, and emergent/critical medical care to wounded and injured service members engaged in active duty. Nurses can work all over the world.

Typical Work Hours and Setting

Armed forces military nurses can work at military bases in the United States or at military bases abroad. The work hours and settings vary according to job position and location.

Education and Training Requirements

- Must be currently licensed as an RN in the United States.
- Most often requires a baccalaureate degree to become a commissioned officer.
- Must possess good interpersonal, listening, and communication skills.
- Should be well disciplined and ready to develop leadership skills.
- Should be free of physical restrictions that impede the ability to provide care in various settings and climates.

Specialty Certification

There is no specialty military nurse certification; however, nurses must apply for a direct commission to obtain a full-time position in the Army, Air Force, or Navy.

Professional Organizations and Online Resources

Army Nursing: http://www.goarmy.com/amedd/nurse.html

Nurse Corps Navy: http://www.navy.com/careers/healthcare/nurse.html#ft-specialties-subspecialties

Air Force Nursing: https://www.airforce.com/careers/specialty-careers/healthcare/careers/nurse

Every Nurse.org: http://everynurse.org/becoming-a-military-nurse/

#39

CARE MANAGER NURSE

Job Description

Care manager nurses monitor patients' overall care in the healthcare system. Many nurses only work with inpatient care management, but some roles make nurses available by phone to assist patients and healthcare teams in outpatient settings. Care managers ensure a seamless transition between care settings, including the facilitation of health information and services between care settings. They can also assist in discharge planning and educating patients and healthcare staff. Some care manager nurses may also engage in quality assurance and utilization review. Care management has been demonstrated to reduce healthcare costs and improve coordination of care and patient care outcomes.

Typical Work Hours and Setting

Most care manager nurses work business hours Monday through Friday. However, some may work evening or weekend hours to facilitate coordination of care.

Education and Training Requirements

- Must be currently licensed as an RN in the United States.
- Most often requires 3 to 5 years of nursing experience; experience in acute care preferred.
- Must possess good interpersonal and communication skills.
- Must have good organizational, analytic, planning, and critical thinking skills.
- Should have a good understanding of health insurance and healthcare reimbursement mechanisms.

Specialty Certification

Nurses can receive board certification as a Certified Managed Care Nurse (CMCN) through the American Board of Managed Care Nursing. To be eligible, nurses must complete curriculum through the American Association of Managed Care Nurses. This includes four components: managed care overview, healthcare economics, healthcare management, and patient issues. Candidates must also submit an application that includes current job description and educational background and preparation.

Professional Organizations and Online Resources

American Association of Managed Care Nurses: http://aamcn.org/

American Board of Managed Care Nursing: http://www.abmcn.org/

National Academy of Certified Care Managers: http://www.naccm.net/

career highlight

Clinical Care Manager

Karol Sue Byers, BS, BSN, RN, CMC

Q: What led you to your current career in nursing?

A: While in community health nursing and also while studying for the BSN, I realized many people struggled with lack of knowledge of the healthcare system and how to maneuver through to obtain services, how those services would be covered, and to understand self-care of their disease or injuries and medications once home. I had also worked in a physician practice and saw that an RN could do so much more there than room patients, take vitals, and assist with procedures. When I became aware of the literature about the patient centered medical home, I realized that was, perhaps, the model of primary care that I had been considering.

Q: What are your typical job duties and responsibilities?

A: In general, the care manager is daily involved with transitions of care, quality metrics, and health education of people with chronic conditions. The care manager is also a leader in the primary care practice as he or she is involved in coaching providers and their staff in practice transformation.

Q: Is there any special training or education required for your job?

A: Some nurses may work as a care manager without training. However, to understand the scope and practice optimally, training is preferred and highly suggested. Training in motivational interviewing, self-determination theory, patient centered medical home, and adult learning theory are some of the aspects of the position which are most useful.

Q: What is the best part of your job?

A: The part of my job that invigorates and gives me joy is the health education and counseling that I am able to offer patients with chronic conditions and seeing them progress in their healthcare goals.

Q: What is the least favorite part of your job?

A: Data tracking and working intensely with quality metrics are the least favorite parts of my job. Those aspects can easily overwhelm the practice aspect, and as company income becomes more important, pressure to work with more data sometimes takes precedence. Also disheartening is observing the primary care practice transformation affecting the physicians and their staff stressfully. The care manager work is somewhat isolating, even though there is coordination between services and patients and with physician and staff contact.

Q: What advice would you give to those interested in pursuing a career in your nursing field?

A: For a nurse interested in pursuing a career in care management, I would advise that he or she obtain at least 2 years' experience in general medical/surgical hospital nursing, as well as experience in clinic or community health/home care and 1 year in utilization. Having a solid background in disease states, medications, community resources, and insurance influence in care is optimal. Also, computer flexibility, as familiarity with electronic medical records (EMRs), Excel, and possibly Access is greatly beneficial. Knowledge of patient centered medical home certification is helpful, as well as care management courses or study.

Q: Anything important that you would like nurses to know about your nursing job?

A: Particular skills needed: organization; leadership toward physicians and office staff as a team member; critical thinking skills; interviewing skills—reflection, motivational interviewing; psychiatric nursing—there's an increasing amount of depression, bipolar conditions, and substance use; ability of the RN to understand himself or herself as a professional working with those of other professions, with the knowledge and understanding of his or her role as defined by the Nurse Practice Act.

#40

CLINICAL RESEARCH NURSE

Job Description

Clinical research nurses engage in all aspects of the research process to make new discoveries and improve medical science and patient care. The duties of a clinical research nurse vary according to specific employer, but typical roles often include recruitment of patients/subjects, obtaining health history/baseline data collection, assessment or collection of physical assessment data or specimens, continual data collection, administration of research interventions, and documenting research-related data and information. The clinical research nurse may also serve as the main contact person between the research subject and the research team.

Typical Work Hours and Setting

Clinical research nurses can work in both inpatient and outpatient settings. They often work in research-intensive medical or academic institutions, governmental agencies, pharmaceutical companies, and private research institutions.

Education and Training Requirements

- Must be currently licensed as an RN in the United States.
- Should possess a baccalaureate degree.
- Most often requires prior clinical experience.
- Must possess good interpersonal, analytic, and communication skills.
- Must have training in the ethical conduct of research.

Specialty Certification

Nurses can obtain board certification through the Association of Clinical Research Professionals. They can obtain a Certified Clinical Research Associate (CCRA) or Certified Clinical Research Coordinator (CCRC) certification.

Professional Organizations and Online Resources

Association of Clinical Research Professionals: http://www.acrpnet.org/

International Association of Clinical Research Nurses: http://iacrn.memberlodge.org/

Society of Clinical Research Associates: https://www.socra.org/

Sigma Theta Tau International Honor Society of Nursing: http://www.nursingsociety.org/

#41

CLINIC NURSE

Job Description

Clinic nursing is one type of nursing in the specialty of ambulatory care. A clinic nurse can work in a variety of outpatient clinics. Clinics can be focused in primary or preventative care, public or community health initiatives, urgent care, outpatient surgery, and other specialty medical care. A clinic nurse utilizes the nursing process in the assessment, implementation, and evaluation of care with clinic patients. Clinic nurses perform and document various assessments, collect blood and other medical specimens, obtain health and medication history, assist with the implementation of specialized procedures, administer medications and treatments, provide patient and family teaching regarding illness/injury management, perform discharges, triage telephone calls, and evaluate patients' response to care.

Typical Work Hours and Setting

Clinic nurses can be employed in a variety of ambulatory outpatient care settings, public and community health departments, managed care practices, and other clinic-based specialty care settings. Hours will vary according to specific employment site. Evening, night, or weekend hours may be required.

Education and Training Requirements

- Must be currently licensed as an RN in the United States.
- Should have 2 to 3 years of medical surgical acute care experience.
- Must possess good interpersonal, listening, and communication skills.
- Should be able to work in a fast-paced environment.
- Must have excellent organizational and prioritization skills.
- Should be able to work as an interdisciplinary team member.

Specialty Certification

There is currently no specific certification for clinic nurses; however, nurses can become nationally certified in ambulatory care and receive the RN-BC designation through the American Nurses Credentialing Center. To be eligible, nurses must have been in practice as a registered nurse for a minimum of 2 years full time, have worked 2,000 hours in ambulatory care and/or telehealth nursing, and have completed 30 hours of continuing education in ambulatory care or telehealth.

Professional Organizations and Online Resources

American Academy of Ambulatory Care Nursing: https://www.aaacn.org/

American Nurses Credentialing Center: http://www.nursecredentialing.org/certification

Ambulatory Surgery Center Association: http://www.ascassociation.org/home

Accreditation Association for Ambulatory Health Care, Inc: http://www.aaahc.org/

42

CRITICAL CARE TRANSPORT FLIGHT NURSE

Job Description

A critical care transport flight nurse, or flight nurse for short, provides in-flight emergency/critical care to patients who have sustained an emergent injury or trauma. A flight nurse must have extensive experience in critical care nursing; that is a mandatory requirement for most positions. They should also have extensive knowledge in basic and advanced life support, mechanical ventilation, and hemodynamic support. Critical care transport flight nurses should be able to work under intense emergent situations and be mentally and physically fit to be able to work in many different environmental conditions.

Typical Work Hours and Setting

Flight nurses can work in both the private (civilian) and military sector. Civilian flight nurses can work for medical flight departments that are part of hospitals or medical centers and fire and other emergency departments. Work hours will vary according to specific employment site.

Education and Training Requirements

- Must be currently licensed as an RN in the United States.
- Must possess a minimum of 3 years (5 years is preferred) of critical care experience in an inpatient intensive care setting.
- Certification in BLS/CPR; ACLS; TNCC/BTLS/PHTLS/TNATC; PALS most often required.
- Must be able to work in an intensive, fast-paced environment and emergent situations.
- Should be free of physical restrictions that can impede the ability to function in various environmental conditions, including in-flight.
- Should be emotionally prepared to witness scenes of intense trauma and accidents.

Specialty Certification

Nurses can become nationally certified as a Certified Flight Registered Nurse (CFRN) through the Board of Certification for Emergency Nursing. To be eligible, nurses must have a current RN license, and 2 years of flight nursing experience is recommended. Nurses may also choose to become certified as a Critical Care Registered Nurse (CCRN) or Certified Emergency Nurse (CEN). Many employers require one of these three specialty certifications as mandatory.

Professional Organizations and Online Resources

Air & Surface Transport Nurses Association: http://astna.org/

Emergency Nurses Association: https://www.ena.org/

Board of Certification for Emergency Nursing: http://www.bcencertifications.org/Get-Certified/CFRN.aspx

American Association of Critical-Care Nurses: http://www.aacn.org/

#43

CRUISE SHIP/ RESORT NURSE

Job Description

A cruise ship/resort nurse provides nursing care to both guests/passengers and cruise ship/resort staff members. Job positions for this type of nursing vary from full time to a seasonal/contract basis. Nurses should have previous knowledge and experience in providing emergency care for injuries and illnesses to patients of all ages. They should be able to work autonomously and independently. Some cruise ship/resort nurses may have other roles and responsibilities in line with some of the duties of occupational health nurses.

Typical Work Hours and Setting

Cruise ship/resort nurses can work in a variety of leisure-associated settings all over the world. This can include cruise ships/luxury liners, riverboat cruises, theme parks, and zoos. Although working in part of a leisure-related setting can appear enticing, nurses must be prepared to encounter a wide variety of patrons, in various emotional states. Nurses should also be prepared to work in various environmental conditions and climates. Hours will vary by specific position.

Education and Training Requirements

- Must be currently licensed as an RN in the United States.
- Requires 3 to 5 years of previous experience as an RN.
- Must possess good interpersonal and communication skills.
- Emergency or occupational health nursing preferred.
- Should be able to work in emergent situations with diverse patients.

Specialty Certification

There is currently no specific certification for cruise ship/resort nurses; however, nurses can become nationally certified in ambulatory care and receive the RN-BC designation through the American Nurses Credentialing Center. To be eligible, nurses must have been in practice as a registered nurse for a minimum of 2 years full time, have worked 2,000 hours in ambulatory care and/or telehealth nursing, and have completed 30 hours of continuing education in ambulatory care or telehealth.

Professional Organizations and Online Resources

American Academy of Ambulatory Care Nursing: https://www.aaacn.org/

American Nurses Credentialing Center: http://www.nursecredentialing.org/certification

Accreditation Association for Ambulatory Health Care, Inc: http://www.aaahc.org/

44

FAITH COMMUNITY NURSE

Job Description

The faith community nurse, otherwise known as a *parish nurse,* provides spiritual support and care for members of a congregation/faith community. Roles and responsibilities may vary but can include preventative education/screenings, counseling, and assessment of patients' holistic healthcare needs. The faith community nurse advocates and assists patients with community and healthcare-associated resources. They also make visits to congregation members who are unable to make it to mass/services or those who are ill and in the hospital or nursing home. Faith community nurses provide emotional and spiritual support to congregation members during religious events such as funerals and baptisms.

Typical Work Hours and Setting

The faith community nurse often works in conjunction with a particular parish or church and assists the clergy with various responsibilities. Work hours and settings can vary but may include travel to congregation members' homes or to hospital settings. Nurses also often provide presence and faith support at baptisms, weddings, or funeral proceedings. Evening and weekend hours should be expected.

Education and Training Requirements

- Must be currently licensed as an RN in the United States.
- Should have strong religious beliefs.
- Must possess excellent interpersonal, listening, and communication skills.
- Should be nonjudgmental, compassionate, and sensitive to patients' concerns.
- Should be able to provide health education teaching and advocate for the health needs of patients/congregation members.

Specialty Certification

Nurses can become nationally certified in faith community nursing and receive the RN-BC designation through the American Nurses Credentialing Center. To be eligible, nurses must submit documentation of their work in, and specialized knowledge and skills related to, faith community nursing. This new mode of certification is done through a portfolio rather than by exam.

Professional Organizations and Online Resources

Church Health Center (formerly the International Parish Nurse Resource Center): http://www.churchhealthcenter.org/forfaithcommunitynurses

Health Ministries Association: http://hmassoc.org/

United Church of Christ: http://www.ucc.org/justice_health_ucc-community-nurses_faith-community-nursehealth

American Nurses Credentialing Center: http://www.nursecredentialing.org/certification

#45

FIRST ASSIST NURSE

Job Description

A first assist nurse, otherwise known as a *registered nurse first assistant* (RNFA), provides nursing care to patients undergoing surgery. They work alongside and provide assistance to surgeons and anesthesiologists in the operating room. Duties can vary but include skills related to the surgery such as direct assistance with suturing, controlling bleeding, administering medications, and monitoring of vital signs. The nurse may also be involved in pre- and post-surgical care of patients, depending on the employment setting. They often provide education regarding the surgery, expectations, postoperative care, and discharge instructions. First assist nurses often provide patients and families with emotional support before and after the surgical procedure.

Typical Work Hours and Setting

A first assist nurse works in both the inpatient and outpatient setting in surgery centers or suites. They can work with any type of surgical specialty. Hours often include evening, night, weekend, and on-call hours.

Education and Training Requirements

- Must be currently licensed as an RN in the United States.
- Most often requires experience working in the perioperative setting prior to becoming an RNFA.
- Must possess excellent interpersonal and communication skills.
- Must be able to work as part of an interdisciplinary team.
- Should be able to work in an intense, high-stress environment.

Specialty Certification

Nurses can become nationally certified as a Certified Registered Nurse First Assistant (CRNFA) through the Competency & Credentialing Institute. Nurses most often need to have the Certified Operating Room Nurse (CNOR) credential in addition to 2,000 hours as a documented registered nurse first assistant.

Professional Organizations and Online Resources

Association of PeriOperative Registered Nurses: http://www.aorn.org/

American Surgical Association: http://americansurgical.org/

Ambulatory Surgery Center Association: http://www.ascassociation.org/home

Competency & Credentialing Institute: http://www.cc-institute.org/crnfa/certification

#46

FORENSIC NURSE

Job Description

Forensic nurses use their nursing skills in the care of patients who are victims of a crime. This includes the collection of physical evidence from patients to be used in the investigation of a crime. They assess patients' injuries and provide medical care and interventions. They also provide emotional support to patients. Forensic nurses provide testimony during criminal trials and may provide consultation services to legal personnel and/or the court system regarding evidence and medical terminology. Forensic nurses should be emotionally prepared to assist patients with injuries from violent crimes.

Typical Work Hours and Setting

Forensic nurses work in settings that provide care for patients who are victims of crimes such as assaults and sexual assaults. Most work in emergency departments or urgent care centers and clinics. Work hours vary but most often include evening, night, and weekend rotations. Nurses may also work long shifts in this position.

Education and Training Requirements

- Must be currently licensed as an RN in the United States.
- Most often requires previous experience in the emergency department.
- Criminal justice or forensics experience preferred.
- Must possess excellent interpersonal, listening, and communication skills.
- Should have excellent skills in data collection and documentation.
- Should be able to provide compassionate and sensitive care to patients who are victims of a crime.

Specialty Certification

There are two specialty certifications available for forensic nurses through the International Association of Forensic Nurses. These include the Sexual Assault Nurse Examiner Adult/Adolescent (SANE-A) and the Sexual Assault Nurse Examiner Pediatric (SANE-P). Nurses can also become certified as an advanced forensic nurse through the American Nurses Credentialing Center, but this requires candidates to have a master's degree. Nurses may also enroll in a forensic nursing training program and earn certification through the American College of Forensic Examiners Institute; however, this option involves additional education.

Professional Organizations and Online Resources

International Association of Forensic Nurses: http://www.forensicnurses.org/

American Forensic Nurses: http://www.amrn.com/

Forensic Nurse Professionals: http://www.fnpi.net/

American Nurses Credentialing Center: http://www.nursecredentialing.org/certification

American College of Forensic Examiners Institute: http://www.acfei.com

#47

INFECTION CONTROL NURSE

Job Description

An infection control nurse works to reduce the spread of infectious diseases in a specific setting or patient population. They can help track and monitor an outbreak and implement strategies to limit or reduce the spread of an infectious agent from developing into epidemic proportions. Nurses provide education and training to other healthcare professionals in the prevention of infections. They also help develop facility-specific policies that prevent or reduce the spread of infections, including isolation and quarantine protocols. Infection control nurses are very knowledgeable and keep abreast of local, state, and national guidelines in place related to infectious disease. They may work closely with public health officials in the event of an outbreak.

Typical Work Hours and Setting

Infection control nurses can work in both inpatient and outpatient settings, both in private healthcare centers and for governmental agencies. Some of these include medical centers, community outreach centers, public health departments, home health agencies, and long-term care facilities. Work hours will vary according to the specific employment agency.

Education and Training Requirements

- Must be currently licensed as an RN in the United States.
- Should possess knowledge in microbiology, epidemiology, or infectious diseases.
- Must possess good interpersonal, listening, and communication skills.
- Should be detail-oriented and be able to collect, analyze, and document infection-control data.
- Must be able to provide education to other members of the healthcare team.
- Must be able to work with other agencies in the tracking and reporting of infectious diseases.

Specialty Certification

Nurses can become nationally certified and receive the Certified Infection Control (CIC) credential through the Certification Board of Infection Control and Epidemiology. To be eligible, nurses must have a baccalaureate degree in nursing and be able to demonstrate competence through a minimum of 2 years work as an RN in infection control.

Professional Organizations and Online Resources

Association for Professionals in Infection Control and Epidemiology: http://www.apic.org/

Centers for Disease Control and Prevention: http://www.cdc.gov/

Infectious Diseases Society of America: https://www.idsociety.org/Index.aspx

Certification Board of Infection Control and Epidemiology, Inc: http://www.cbic.org/

#48

INFORMATICS NURSE

Job Description

Informatics in healthcare is an emerging field. The informatics nurse is the liaison between medical staff and information systems/medical technology. They are knowledgeable and skilled in the functioning, use, and maintenance of healthcare information systems. In addition to providing training and support to system users, they may engage in policy writing, special projects, the development of new or modifications to protocols related to information systems, and the oversight of patch management of information systems.

Typical Work Hours and Setting

Informatics nurses can work in any inpatient or outpatient setting where medical technology exists. The work setting may require travel to satellite offices or facilities to train staff. Hours are normally business hours, daytime Monday through Friday; however, some evening or weekend hours may be required.

Education and Training Requirements

- Must be currently licensed as an RN in the United States.
- Most often requires experience or a degree in information systems.
- Must possess excellent verbal and written communication skills.
- Must be knowledgeable with various forms of information technology.
- Should be able to educate healthcare staff in the use of various forms of medical technology and information systems.

Specialty Certification

Nurses can become nationally certified as an informatics nurse and earn the RN-BC designation through the American Nurses Credentialing Center. To be eligible, nurses must have a baccalaureate degree in nursing or another relevant field, have 2 years minimum practice as an RN, with 2,000 hours in informatics nursing within the past 3 years. Additionally, eligible candidates must have 30 hours of continuing education in informatics within the last 3 years.

Professional Organizations and Online Resources

American Nursing Informatics Association: https://www.ania.org/

Alliance for Nursing Informatics: http://www.allianceni.org/

American Medical Informatics Association: https://www.amia.org/

Healthcare Information and Management Systems Society: https://www.himss.org/

American Nurses Credentialing Center: http://www.nursecredentialing.org/certification

#49

INFUSION SPECIALIST NURSE

Job Description

An infusion specialist nurse administers medication and fluids to patients intravenously. They are specialized in starting/monitoring/discontinuing intravenous lines. They monitor patients during infusions for complications or reactions and manage care of the equipment used, such as tubing, medication and fluid bags, and needles. Infusion nurses assess patients' general and vascular health and response to infusion treatment. They provide patients with education regarding illness, infusion therapy, and discharge instructions. They are also excellent resources for other nursing and healthcare staff and are often called to provide assistance with troubleshooting of infusion-related issues and/or assist with starting venous access lines.

Typical Work Hours and Setting

Infusion specialist nurses can work in both inpatient and outpatient settings. They can work in ambulatory infusion centers, cancer/chemotherapy clinics, physician offices, home health agencies, and ambulatory surgery centers. Hours vary according to the clinical site of employment.

Education and Training Requirements

- Must be currently licensed as an RN in the United States.
- Most often requires previous medical surgical or acute care experience as an RN.
- Must possess good interpersonal, listening, and communication skills.
- Must have excellent skills related to management of intravenous therapy.
- Should be able to provide comfort and support to patients who are fearful of receiving intravenous therapy.

Specialty Certification

Nurses can become nationally certified and earn the Certified Registered Nurse Infusion (CRNI) through the Infusion Nurses Society. To be eligible to sit for the exam, nurses must have an active RN license and a minimum of 1,600 hours of experience in infusion therapy as an RN.

Professional Organizations and Online Resources

Infusion Nurses Society: https://www.ins1.org/default.aspx

National Home Infusion Association: http://www.nhia.org/

Association for Vascular Access: http://www.avainfo.org/

Vascular Access Society of the Americas: http://www.vasamd.org/

#50

LEGAL NURSE CONSULTANT

Job Description

A legal nurse consultant is a registered nurse who is an important part of the litigation team. Their role is to examine, analyze, and report informed opinions about health-related legal cases that fall within the medical-legal scope. This can include cases related to personal injury, medical malpractice, workers' compensation, billing fraud, etc. Legal nurse consultants utilize their nursing and healthcare experience to make determinations based on the documentation and evidence provided regarding malpractice related to the medical care event. They fill the gap between healthcare and the law.

Typical Work Hours and Setting

Legal nurse consultants can find employment within law firms and offices or can work on a contract-to-contract basis. They may find employment at insurance companies or governmental agencies. Some legal nurse consultants provide consulting work on the side as an addition to their full-time position, while others have their own consulting business.

Education and Training Requirements

- Must be currently licensed as an RN in the United States.
- Should have at least 5 years experience working in medical surgical or critical care.
- Must possess good analytic and communication skills.
- Must be able to provide unbiased and thorough documentation of the results of their analysis.
- Previous legal experience is not necessary; however, there are programs in legal nurse consulting available.

Specialty Certification

Nurses can become nationally certified and earn the Legal Nurse Consultant Certified (LNCC) credential through the American Association of Legal Nurse Consultants Certification Board. To be eligible, nurses must have a current RN license, a minimum of 5 years practice as an RN, and a minimum of 2,000 hours of legal nurse consulting experience within the past 5 years.

Professional Organizations and Online Resources

American Association of Legal Nurse Consultants: http://www.aalnc.org/

National Alliance of Certified Legal Nurse Consultants: http://www.legalnurse.com/certified-legal-nurse-consultants/naclnc-association/naclnc-association-membership

American Nurses Association: http://www.nursingworld.org/

#51

MASSAGE THERAPY NURSE

Job Description

Massage therapy nurses are registered nurses that have also been trained in massage therapy. Nurses can specialize in medical massage, therapeutic massage, or both. Many massage therapy nurses work in health spas or wellness facilities, while others work independently as consultants or have their own nurse massage businesses. Using massage, nurses promote holistic healing using a variety of techniques and approaches. Nurses focus on the health of both mind and body and the unique healing power of massage through the techniques they employ.

Typical Work Hours and Setting

Massage therapy nurses can work at health or beauty spas, chiropractor offices, or massage therapy offices. They can also work independently (depending on state regulations) or as a consultant.

Education and Training Requirements

- Must be currently licensed as an RN in the United States.
- Must have licensure/training (state dependent) in massage therapy.
- Must possess good interpersonal and communication skills.
- Should be able to provide sensitive and holistic care to a variety of clients.
- Should be free of physical restrictions that can impede the ability to perform various types of massage.

Specialty Certification

Nurses who have received training in a massage therapy program can apply for the national certification examination in massage therapy through the National Certification Board for Therapeutic Massage and Bodywork (NCBTMB). Each state has its own regulations governing whether a license is required to practice certain types of massage therapy. Check with your individual state for details.

Professional Organizations and Online Resources

National Association of Nurse Massage Therapists: http://www.nanmt.org/

National Certification Board for Therapeutic Massage and Bodywork: http://www.ncbtmb.org/

American Massage Therapy Association: https://www.amtamassage.org/index.html

National Association of Massage Therapists: http://namtonline.com/

Massage Therapy Foundation: http://mtf.amtamassage.org/

52

MISSIONARY NURSE

Job Description

A missionary nurse provides nursing care to patients in need across various regions of the world. Nurses often need to travel to underdeveloped nations and areas that are lacking in the basic necessities required to support life. Often, missionary work focuses on providing assistance to children and families following a natural disaster or in times of war. Nurses focus on providing holistic care that includes physical, psychological, social, and spiritual domains.

Typical Work Hours and Setting

Missionary nurses work as part of churches and religious congregations and humanitarian and nonprofit groups to travel to various regions around the world to provide missionary work. Nurses often have another permanent nursing position at which they work when they are not involved with missionary work.

Education and Training Requirements

- Must be currently licensed as an RN in the United States.
- Most often requires some experience in nursing care.
- Must possess good interpersonal, listening, and communication skills.
- Ability to speak a foreign language(s) may be beneficial.
- Should be willing to travel and function in various extreme climates or in locations that may be dangerous.

Specialty Certification

There is no specialty certification for missionary nurses at this time. Nurses who are part of faith communities can choose to become certified as a faith community nurse and receive the RN-BC designation through the American Nurses Credentialing Center. To be eligible, nurses must submit documentation of their work in, and specialized knowledge and skills related to, faith community nursing. This new mode of certification is done through a portfolio rather than by exam.

Professional Organizations and Online Resources

Nurses for the Nations:
http://www.nursesforthenations.org/

Samaritan's Purse World Medical Mission:
https://www.samaritanspurse.org/

Nurses Christian Fellowship: http://ncf-jcn.org/
resources/missions

National Association of Catholic Nurses USA:
https://nacn-usa.org/

#53

NURSE AUTHOR

Job Description

A nurse author is a registered nurse who also writes and publishes his or her work in the form of a book, medical journal, professional organizations, or freelance. Although work is typically focused in healthcare and utilized for the purposes of education, research, or training, nurse authors can also write historical pieces, biographies, and fiction/novels. Nurse authors can also contribute to manuscripts for speeches involving healthcare details or to television scripts. Most nurse authors write publications for healthcare-related materials that are based on their prior clinical experience in the healthcare setting.

Typical Work Hours and Setting

A nurse author can work for a publishing company or as part of a medical journal board. Most nurse authors write and publish material that is not part of their regular nursing job and is in addition to the scope of their usual nursing position requirements. Work hours vary according to specific writing job/project.

Education and Training Requirements

- Must be currently licensed as an RN in the United States.
- Must have excellent written communication skills.
- Must be able to meet deadlines for submitting work for publication.
- Should be familiar with various professional writing styles (APA, AMA, MLA).
- Should be familiar with the publication/publishing process.

Specialty Certification

There is no specialty certification for nurse authors specifically; however, there is a credential for Medical Writer Certified (MWC) that is available through the American Medical Writers Association. To be eligible, candidates must have a bachelor's degree in any discipline and a minimum of 2 years full-time work experience within the past 5 years.

Professional Organizations and Online Resources

American Medical Writers Association: http://www.amwa.org/

Nurse Author & Editor: http://naepub.com/

International Academy of Nursing Editors: https://nursingeditors.com/

Sigma Theta Tau International Honor Society of Nursing: http://www.nursingsociety.org/

#54

NURSE CONSULTANT

Job Description

A nurse consultant is a registered nurse who provides a healthcare/nursing-related service, contribution, or act to another entity. Most often healthcare-related, the nurse consultant uses his or her previous experience in nursing to solve a problem, provide a service, or meet a need for a third party. Examples of nurse consultant work can include consultation on legal matters and issues (see #50: Legal Nurse Consultant), protocols for healthcare-related interventions, knowledge of the healthcare process and insurance, specialized knowledge in an illness or other medical specialty, specialized knowledge regarding a patient care population, and knowledge of medical devices/equipment.

Typical Work Hours and Setting

Work hours will vary and depend on the specific consultant role. Some consultant positions are temporary and on a contract-to-contract basis. Others involve travel and time that may or may not be compensated. Nurse consultants must be able to negotiate compensation for their contribution.

Education and Training Requirements

- Must be currently licensed as an RN in the United States.
- Should have a baccalaureate degree.
- Must be savvy with business and economics.
- Should have excellent organizational, planning, negotiation, and marketing skills.
- Should be comfortable selling oneself and with public speaking.
- Should be willing to travel for consulting jobs and new business ventures.
- Should have the ability to work with others to carry out a business plan.

Specialty Certification

There is no specialty certification for a nurse consultant, businessperson, or entrepreneur.

Professional Organizations and Online Resources

National Nurses in Business Association:
https://nnbanow.com/nurse-consultant-faq/

American Nurses Association:
http://www.nursingworld.org/

#55

NURSE EDUCATOR

Job Description

A nurse educator teaches the learner healthcare-related material in a variety of contexts and settings. This can include educating students in academic nursing programs within colleges and universities, educating and training unlicensed medical and nursing assistants and home health aides, and providing orientation and training to licensed nursing personnel, including RNs and LPNs. Nurse educators deliver education regarding medical and nursing knowledge and skills and evaluate to see whether learning objectives were met. The nurse educator uses a variety of teaching modalities and should be knowledgeable about course development, lecture design, test development, item writing, and information systems used in the delivery of academic courses or healthcare orientation training programs.

Typical Work Hours and Setting

Nurse educators can work in academic institutions, inpatient and outpatient healthcare facilities, and in public/community health. Nurse educators teaching in the clinical setting may work early or late shifts. Nurse educators in healthcare institutions work hours that may vary and also may include work in evenings, nights, or weekends to provide education and training to all staff.

Education and Training Requirements

- Must be currently licensed as an RN in the United States.
- Most often requires a master's degree if teaching at the academic level. Nurses may be able to work as educators within some healthcare institutions with a baccalaureate degree or as clinical adjunct faculty.
- Must possess excellent interpersonal and verbal and written communication skills.
- Education experience is recommended.
- Should be comfortable and effective with public speaking.
- Should be able to verbalize and teach content using a variety of teaching methods to diverse learners.

Specialty Certification

Nurses can become nationally certified as a nurse educator earning the Certification for Nurse Educator (CNE) credential through the National League for Nursing. To be eligible, nurses must have a current RN license, have their master's degree in nursing or higher, and 2 years full-time work as a nurse educator in an academic nursing program within the past 5 years.

Professional Organizations and Online Resources

National League for Nursing: http://www.nln.org/

Professional Nurse Educators Group: https://pneg.org/

Association for Nursing Professional Development: http://www.anpd.org/

American Association of Colleges of Nursing: http://www.aacn.nche.edu/

56

NURSE MANAGER

Job Description

A nurse manager is a registered nurse who oversees the operations of a specific patient care unit, center, or healthcare-related setting. Most nurse managers have primarily administrative roles and often do not engage in clinical practice. Their main responsibilities include interviewing/hiring new employees; monitoring unit staffing; completing performance evaluations for employees; oversight of budgets; implementation of policies; adhering to institution, state, and federal regulations; providing leadership for the unit; oversight of quality initiatives on the unit; and being a liaison between staff and upper management.

Typical Work Hours and Setting

A nurse manager can find a position in both the inpatient and outpatient setting. Although many manager positions involve a Monday through Friday business hours schedule, most managers are required to provide 24/7 support for their designated unit or care setting.

Education and Training Requirements

- Must be currently licensed as an RN in the United States.
- Most often requires several years of nursing experience in the care setting.
- Must possess good interpersonal, listening, and communication skills.
- Must be able to provide leadership and management to the team.
- Should be a people person who enjoys taking charge and leading his or her team members.

Specialty Certification

Nurses can obtain the credential as a Certified Nurse Manager Leader (CNML) through the American Association of Critical-Care Nurses Certification Corporation or a Certified in Executive Nursing Practice (CENP) through the American Organization of Nurse Executives Credentialing Center.

Professional Organizations and Online Resources

American Organization of Nurse Executives: http://www.aone.org/

American Organization of Nurse Executives Credentialing Center: http://www.aone.org/activities/certification.shtml

American Association of Critical-Care Nurses Certification Corporation: http://www.aacn.org/dm/mainpages/certificationhome.aspx?menu=certification

National Association of Directors of Nursing Administration in Long Term Care: https://www.nadona.org/

#57

QUALITY COMPLIANCE NURSE

Job Description

A quality compliance, or assurance, nurse is a registered nurse who works to ensure that quality is maintained in the healthcare setting. Quality assurance or compliance can be related to just about anything within the scope of the healthcare system. This can include patient care; staffing/employees; billing and insurance; county, state, and federal regulations; documentation; information systems/electronic medical records; and systems-related policies and procedures. Although this is broad, each quality compliance nurse position may differ in terms of specific roles and responsibilities. They are important members of the healthcare system in ensuring that compliance and regulations are met and that the system is at optimal functioning in the provision of cost-effective quality care.

Typical Work Hours and Setting

Quality compliance nurses can work in both the inpatient and outpatient setting. They can work in medical centers, medical practices, managed care, home healthcare, public and community health, hospices, and in long-term care. Hours will vary but are mostly during business hours Monday through Friday.

Education and Training Requirements

- Must be currently licensed as an RN in the United States.
- Most often requires at least 5 years of clinical experience as a registered nurse.
- Must possess good analytic and documentation skills.
- Should have a good knowledge of various healthcare-related information systems and documentation systems.
- Should be detail-oriented and able to meet deadlines.

Specialty Certification

Nurses can become a Certified Professional in Healthcare Quality and earn the CPHQ credential through the National Association for Healthcare Quality. To be eligible, nurses should have a current RN license and have worked full time in healthcare quality for a minimum of 2 years.

Professional Organizations and Online Resources

National Association for Healthcare Quality: http://www.nahq.org/

Healthcare Compliance Association: http://www.hcca-info.org/AboutHCCA/AboutHCCA.aspx

Agency for Healthcare Research and Quality: http://www.ahrq.gov/

#58

PAIN MANAGEMENT NURSE

Job Description

A pain management nurse has specialized knowledge and skills in all aspects of pain management. This includes utilizing the nursing process in the care of patients who are living with pain from a variety of conditions. The pain management nurse is an expert in pain assessment, management, and evaluation. They deliver nursing and medical interventions for the management of pain, which can include both pharmacological and non-pharmacological therapies. The goal of the pain management nurse is to assist patients with strategies that reduce or remove their pain so they can engage in activities of daily living, which can improve their overall quality of life.

Typical Work Hours and Setting

Pain management nurses can work in both inpatient and outpatient care settings. This can include pain management clinics or centers, oncology practices, radiation therapy, hospice and palliative care, ambulatory surgery centers, rehabilitation facilities, home healthcare, and long-term care facilities. Hours will vary according to the employment site.

Education and Training Requirements

- Must be currently licensed as an RN in the United States.
- Most often requires previous acute care experience.
- Must possess good interpersonal, listening, and communication skills.
- Should provide sensitive and compassionate care to patients of all ages.
- Must be able to provide culturally competent care.
- Should have advanced knowledge in the pharmacological and non-pharmacological management of pain.

Specialty Certification

Nurses can become nationally certified in pain management nursing and earn the RN-BC credential through the American Nurses Credentialing Center. To be eligible, nurses must have a minimum of 2 years of full-time experience as an RN, a minimum of 2,000 hours working in pain management in the past 3 years, and 30 hours of continuing education with 15 hours in pain management within the past 3 years.

Professional Organizations and Online Resources

American Society for Pain Management Nursing: http://www.aspmn.org/Pages/default.aspx

American Chronic Pain Association: https://theacpa.org/

American Academy of Pain Management: http://www.aapainmanage.org/

American Nurses Credentialing Center: http://www.nursecredentialing.org/

#59

RURAL HEALTH NURSE

Job Description

A rural health nurse provides general nursing care to patients of all ages who reside in rural or remote regions. Although rural nurses can be specialized, most have a broad medical knowledge base and an excellent understanding of the developmental stages, as patients can be any age along the life span. They should be very knowledgeable about the people, culture, and region they are providing care to, including community resources available. Rural health nurses should be able to provide health-related information about illness prevention and management to patients and their families.

Typical Work Hours and Setting

Rural health nurses can work in both inpatient and outpatient settings within rural health. This can include working at clinics or medical facilities that provide care to individuals living in rural settings, home health or public healthcare, and primary care. Travel to remote rural regions should be expected.

Education and Training Requirements

- Must be currently licensed as an RN in the United States.
- Most often requires 3 to 5 years of experience in medical surgical nursing or primary care.
- Must possess good interpersonal, listening, and communication skills.
- Should be willing to travel to remote areas in various climates and weather.
- Should be able to establish good rapport and nurse-patient relationships with patients.

Specialty Certification

Currently, there is no specialty certification available for rural nursing. Nurses can pursue specialty certification in medical-surgical nursing, general nursing practice, or ambulatory care nursing and earn the RN-BC designation through the American Nurses Credentialing Center.

Professional Organizations and Online Resources

Rural Nurse Organization: http://www.rno.org/

National Rural Health Association: http://www.ruralhealthweb.org/

National Rural Health Resource Center: https://www.ruralcenter.org/

#60

TRAVEL NURSE

Job Description

A travel nurse is a registered nurse who travels to various locations to work in a healthcare setting for a limited amount of time. Travel nurse assignments can range from 13 to 26 weeks per assignment. Travel nurses are always needed due to the shortages of nurses in the country, so they have flexibility in the assignments that they choose. Travel nurses can have a broad general nursing knowledge in medical-surgical or can specialize in a particular domain. Wages for travel nurses are competitive, and housing/travel expenses are paid for as part of the job.

Typical Work Hours and Setting

Travel nurses have great flexibility in the assignments that they choose and can explore any area of the country they want through their job as a travel nurse. Travel nurses can work in both inpatient and outpatient settings in acute and chronic care. Hours and schedule will vary according to job contract and can include any shifts, holidays, and weekends.

Education and Training Requirements

- Must be currently licensed as an RN in the United States.
- Most often requires 3 to 5 years of prior nursing experience.
- Must possess good interpersonal, listening, and communication skills.
- Should enjoy travel and be receptive to moving frequently for the next assignment.

Specialty Certification

Although there is no specialty certification specifically for travel nursing, many travel nurses obtain specialty certification in their respected specialty. Travel nurses who have board or national certification are more attractive candidates for travel nurse positions.

Professional Organizations and Online Resources

American Travel Health Nurses Association:
http://www.athna.org/

National Association of Travel Healthcare Organizations:
http://www.natho.org/

Travel Nursing Central:
http://www.travelnursingcentral.com/

American Nurses Association:
http://www.nursingworld.org/

APPENDIX

NON-HOSPITAL NURSING SPECIALTY WEBSITES AND RESOURCES

A

Accreditation Association for Ambulatory Health Care, Inc:
http://www.aaahc.org/

Agency for Healthcare Research and Quality:
http://www.ahrq.gov/

Air & Surface Transport Nurses Association: http://astna.org/

Air Force Nursing: https://www.airforce.com/careers/specialty-careers/healthcare/careers/nurse

Alliance for Nursing Informatics: http://www.allianceni.org/

Ambulatory Surgery Center Association:
http://www.ascassociation.org/home

American Academy of Ambulatory Care Nursing:
https://www.aaacn.org/

American Academy of Ambulatory Care Nursing Telehealth: https://www.aaacn.org/telehealth

American Academy of Child & Adolescent Psychiatry: http://www.aacap.org/

American Academy of Dermatology: https://www.aad.org/

American Academy of Hospice and Palliative Medicine: http://aahpm.org/

American Academy of Pain Management: http://www.aapainmanage.org/

American Academy of Pediatrics: https://www.aap.org/

American Assisted Living Nurses Association: https://www.alnursing.org/

American Association for Geriatric Psychiatry: http://www.aagponline.org/

American Association of Cardiovascular and Pulmonary Rehabilitation: https://www.aacvpr.org/

American Association of Colleges of Nursing: http://www.aacn.nche.edu/

American Association of Critical-Care Nurses: http://www.aacn.org/

American Association of Critical-Care Nurses Certification Corporation: http://www.aacn.org/dm/mainpages/certificationhome.aspx?menu=certification

American Association of Diabetes Educators: https://www.diabeteseducator.org/

American Association of Heart Failure Nurses: http://www.aahfn.org/

American Association of Legal Nurse Consultants: http://www.aalnc.org/

American Association of Managed Care Nurses:
http://aamcn.org/

American Association of Occupational Health Nurses:
http://aaohn.org/

American Association on Intellectual and Developmental
Disabilities: https://aaidd.org/

American Board for Occupational Health Nurses, Inc:
https://www.abohn.org/

American Board of Cardiovascular Medicine:
http://www.abcmcertification.com/

American Board of Dermatology: https://www.abderm.org/

American Board of Genetic Counseling: http://www.abgc.net/

American Board of Managed Care Nursing:
http://www.abmcn.org/

American Camp Association: http://www.acacamps.org/

American Case Management Association:
http://www.acmaweb.org/

American Chronic Pain Association: https://theacpa.org/

American College Health Association: http://www.acha.org/

American College of Forensic Examiners Institute:
http://www.acfei.com

American Correctional Association: http://www.aca.org/

American Correctional Health Services Association:
http://www.achsa.org/

American Diabetes Association: http://www.diabetes.org/

American Forensic Nurses: http://www.amrn.com/

American Geriatrics Society:
http://www.americangeriatrics.org/

American Heart Association:
http://www.heart.org/HEARTORG/

American Massage Therapy Association:
https://www.amtamassage.org/index.html

American Medical Informatics Association:
https://www.amia.org/

American Medical Writers Association:
http://www.amwa.org/

American Nephrology Nurses Association:
https://www.annanurse.org/

American Nurses Association:
http://www.nursingworld.org/

American Nurses Credentialing Center:
http://www.nursecredentialing.org/certification

American Nursing Informatics Association:
https://www.ania.org/

American Organization of Nurse Executives:
http://www.aone.org/

American Organization of Nurse Executives Credentialing
Center: http://www.aone.org/activities/certification.shtml

American Psychiatric Nurses Association:
http://www.apna.org/

American Public Health Association: https://www.apha.org/

American School Health Association:
http://www.ashaweb.org/

American Society for Pain Management Nursing:
http://www.aspmn.org/pages/default.aspx

American Society for Therapeutic Radiation Oncology:
https://www.astro.org/home/

American Society of Addiction Medicine: http://www.asam.org/

American Surgical Association: http://americansurgical.org/

American Telemedicine Association: http://www.americantelemed.org/

American Travel Health Nurses Association: http://www.athna.org/

American Urological Association: https://www.auanet.org/

Army Nursing: http://www.goarmy.com/amedd/nurse.html

Association for Addiction Professionals: http://www.naadac.org/

Association for Nursing Professional Development: http://www.anpd.org/

Association for Professionals in Infection Control and Epidemiology: http://www.apic.org/

Association for Radiologic & Imaging Nursing: http://arinursing.org/

Association for Vascular Access: http://www.avainfo.org/

Association of Camp Nurses: http://www.acn.org/

Association of Clinical Research Professionals: http://www.acrpnet.org/

Association of Community Health Nursing Educators: http://www.achne.org/

Association of Occupational Health Professionals in Health-care: https://www.aohp.org/

Association of Pediatric Hematology/Oncology Nurses: http://www.aphon.org/

Association of PeriOperative Registered Nurses: http://www.aorn.org/

Association of Professional Developmental Disabilities Administrators: http://www.apdda.org/

Association of Public Health Nurses: http://www.phnurse.org/

Association of Rehabilitation Nurses: http://www.rehabnurse.org/

B

Bemidji State University Camp Nursing Certificate: http://www.bemidjistate.edu/academics/graduate-studies/programs/camp-nursing/

Board of Certification for Emergency Nursing: http://www.bcencertifications.org/

Board of Nephrology Examiners Nursing Technology: http://www.bonent.org/

C

Camp Nurse Jobs.com: http://www.campnursejobs.com/

Case Management Society of America: http://www.cmsa.org/

Centers for Disease Control and Prevention: http://www.cdc.gov/

Certification Board for Urologic Nurses and Associates: https://www.cbuna.org/

Certification Board of Infection Control and Epidemiology, Inc: http://www.cbic.org/

Childbirth and Postpartum Professional Association: http://www.cappa.net/

Childbirth Professionals International: http://thechildbirthprofession.com/

Church Health Center (formerly International Parish Nurse Resource Center): http://www.churchhealthcenter.org/forfaithcommunitynurses

Commission for Case Manager Certification: https://ccmcertification.org/

Competency & Credentialing Institute: http://www.cc-institute.org/crnfa/certification

Correctional Nurse.net: http://correctionalnurse.net/

D

Dermatology Nurses' Association: http://www.dnanurse.org/

Developmental Disabilities Nurses Association: https://ddna.org/

DiabetesNet.com: http://www.diabetesnet.com/

E

Emergency Nurses Association: https://www.ena.org/

End of Life Nursing Education Consortium (ELNEC) Pediatric Palliative Care: http://www.aacn.nche.edu/elnec/about/pediatric-palliative-care

Every Nurse.org: http://everynurse.org/becoming-a-military-nurse/

F

Forensic Nurse Professionals: http://www.fnpi.net/

G

Genomic Careers: https://www.genome.gov/genomiccareers/career.cfm?id=22

Gerontological Society of America: https://www.geron.org/

H

Health Ministries Association: http://hmassoc.org/

Healthcare Compliance Association: http://www.hcca-info.org/aboutHCCA/aboutHCCA.aspx

Healthcare Information and Management Systems Society: https://www.himss.org/

Hospice & Palliative Credentialing Center: http://hpcc.advancingexpertcare.org/

Hospice & Palliative Credentialing Center CHPPN Certification: http://hpcc.advancingexpertcare.org/competence/rn-peds-chppn/

Hospice & Palliative Nurses Association: http://hpna.advancingexpertcare.org/

I

Infectious Diseases Society of America: https://www.idsociety.org/Index.aspx

Infusion Nurses Society: https://www.ins1.org/default.aspx

Initiative for Pediatric Palliative Care: http://www.ippcweb.org/

Institute of Pediatric Nursing: http://www.ipedsnursing.org/ptisite/control/index

International Academy of Nursing Editors: https://nursingeditors.com/

International Association of Clinical Research Nurses: http://iacrn.memberlodge.org/

International Association of Forensic Nurses: http://www.forensicnurses.org/

International Association of Rehabilitation Professionals: http://www.rehabpro.org/

International Board of Lactation Consultant Examiners:
http://iblce.org/

International Childbirth Education Association:
http://icea.org/

International Continence Society: http://www.ics.org/

International Lactation Consultant Association:
http://www.ilca.org/home

International Nurses Society on Addictions:
http://www.intnsa.org/certification

International Society for Telemedicine and eHealth:
https://www.isfteh.org/

International Society of Nurses in Cancer Care:
http://www.isncc.org/

International Society of Nurses in Genetics:
http://www.isong.org/

International Society of Psychiatric-Mental Health Nurses:
http://www.ispn-psych.org/

L

Lactation Education Resources:
https://www.lactationtraining.com/

Leading Age (formerly American Association of Homes and
Services for the Aging): http://www.leadingage.org/

M

Massage Therapy Foundation: http://mtf.amtamassage.org/

Maternal-Child Health Nurse Leadership Academy:
http://www.nursingsociety.org/learn-grow/leadership-
institute/maternal-child-health-nurse-leadership-academy

N

National Academy of Certified Care Managers:
http://www.naccm.net/

National Alliance of Certified Legal Nurse Consultants:
http://www.legalnurse.com/certified-legal-nurse-consultants/naclnc-association/naclnc-association-membership

National Association for Healthcare Quality:
http://www.nahq.org/

National Association for Home Care & Hospice:
http://www.nahc.org/

National Association for the Support of Long Term Care:
https://www.nasl.org/

National Association of Addiction Treatment Providers:
https://www.naatp.org/

National Association of Catholic Nurses USA:
https://nacn-usa.org/

National Association of Directors of Nursing Administration in Long Term Care: https://www.nadona.org/

National Association of Massage Therapists:
http://namtonline.com/

National Association of Nurse Massage Therapists:
http://www.nanmt.org/

National Association of Pediatric Nurse Practitioners:
https://www.napnap.org/

National Association of School Nurses:
http://www.nasn.org/

National Association of Travel Healthcare Organizations:
http://www.natho.org/

National Board for Certification of School Nurses:
http://www.nbcsn.org/

National Board of Public Health Examiners:
https://www.nbphe.org/

National Center for Assisted Living:
https://www.ahcancal.org/ncal/pages/index.aspx

National Center on Domestic Violence, Trauma & Mental
Health: http://www.nationalcenterdvtraumamh.org/

National Certification Board for Diabetes Educators:
http://www.ncbde.org/

National Certification Board for Therapeutic Massage and
Bodywork: http://www.ncbtmb.org/

National Commission on Correctional Health Care:
http://www.ncchc.org/

National Gerontological Nursing Association:
http://www.ngna.org/

National Home Infusion Association: http://www.nhia.org/

National Hospice and Palliative Care Organization:
http://www.nhpco.org/

National Hospice and Palliative Care Organization Pediatric:
http://www.nhpco.org/pediatric

National Kidney Foundation: https://www.kidney.org/

National League for Nursing: http://www.nln.org/

National Long Term Care Network: http://nltcn.com/

National Nurses in Business Association:
https://nnbanow.com/nurse-consultant-faq/

National Registered Nurse Case Manager Training Center:
https://nationalrncasemanagertraining.com/welcome/

National Rehabilitation Association:
https://www.nationalrehab.org/

National Resource Center on Domestic Violence:
http://www.nrcdv.org/dvrn/

National Rural Health Association:
http://www.ruralhealthweb.org/

National Rural Health Resource Center:
https://www.ruralcenter.org/

National Society of Genetics Counselors:
http://www.nsgc.org/

Nephrology Nursing Certification Commission:
https://www.nncc-exam.org/

Nurse Author & Editor: http://naepub.com/

Nurse Corps Navy: http://www.navy.com/careers/
healthcare/nurse.html#ft-specialties-subspecialties

Nurses Christian Fellowship:
http://ncf-jcn.org/resources/missions

Nurses for the Nations: http://www.nursesforthenations.org/

O

Oncology Nursing Society: https://www.ons.org/

Oncology Nursing Certification Corporation:
http://www.oncc.org/

P

Pediatric Nursing Certification Board:
https://www.pncb.org/ptistore/control/exams/pn/index

Prepared Childbirth Educators, Inc:
https://www.childbirtheducation.org/

Preventive Cardiovascular Nurses Association:
http://pcna.net/

Professional Nurse Educators Group: https://pneg.org/

Psychiatric Nursing.com:
http://www.psychiatricnursing.com/home

Q

Quad Council Coalition: http://www.quadcouncilphn.org/

R

Radiologic Nursing Certification Board:
https://www.certifiedradiologynurse.org

Rural Nurse Organization: http://www.rno.org/

S

Samaritan's Purse World Medical Mission:
https://www.samaritanspurse.org/

School Nurse.com:
http://www.schoolnurse.com/public/department42.cfm

Sigma Theta Tau International Honor Society of Nursing:
http://www.nursingsociety.org/

Society of Clinical Research Associates:
https://www.socra.org/

Society of Interventional Radiology: http://www.sirweb.org/

Society of Urologic Nurses and Associates:
https://www.suna.org/

T

Telemedicine Nursing Fact Sheet:
http://www.americantelemed.org/docs/default-document-library/fact_sheet_final.pdf?sfvrsn=2

Travel Nursing Central:
http://www.travelnursingcentral.com/

U

United Church of Christ: http://www.ucc.org/justice_health_ucc-community-nurses_faith-community-nursehealth

United Spinal Association: http://www.spinalcord.org/

United States Lactation Consultant Association:
https://uslca.org/

Urology Care Foundation: http://www.urologyhealth.org/

V

Vascular Access Society of the Americas:
http://www.vasamd.org/

W

Wound, Ostomy and Continence Nurses Society:
http://www.wocn.org/

Wound, Ostomy and Continence Nursing Certification Board:
https://www.wocncb.org/

INDEX

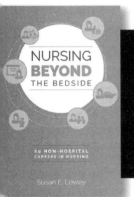 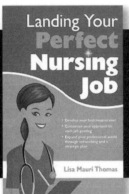 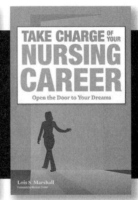 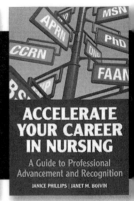

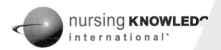

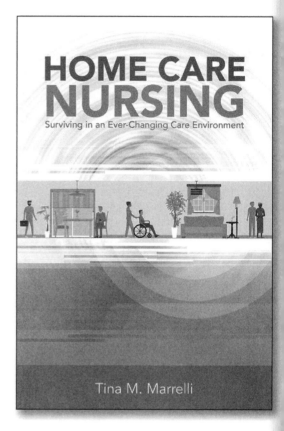
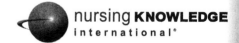